MW00352222

Essential Guide To
MACROBIOTICS

Carl Ferré

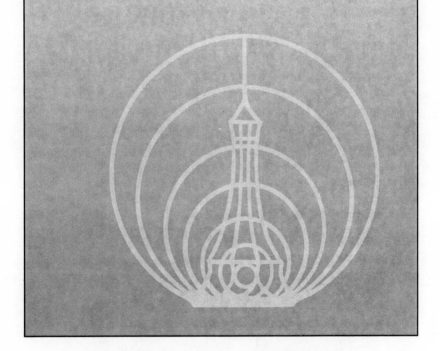

**Newly revised and expanded version of
Pocket Guide to Macrobiotics**

George Ohsawa Macrobiotic Foundation
Chico, California

This book would not have been possible without the help of many people. I give my sincere thanks to my family for their much-needed love and support; to my macrobiotic teahers, Herman and Cornellia Aihara, George and Lima Ohsawa, and Michio and Aveline Kushi; to my colleagues and fellow workers Sandy Rothman, Laurel and Bob Ruggles, and Bob and Kathy Ligon; to at all those who have called or come by with a question or an answer.

Other Books of Carl Ferré
Acid Alkaline Companion
Essential Ohsawa (editor)

Keyboarding by Alice Salinero
Copy editing by Kathy Keller
Cover design by Carl Campbell
Text layout and design by Carl Ferré

First Edition	1997
Current Printing: edited and reformatted	2011 Oct 1

© copyright 2011, 1997 by
George Ohsawa Macrobiotic Foundation
 PO Box 3998, Chico, California 95927-3998
 530-566-9765; fax 530-566-9768; *gomf@earthlink.net*
 www.ohsawamacrobiotics.com

Published with the help of East West Center for Macrobiotics
 www.eastwestmacrobiotics.com

ISBN 978-0-918860-66-8

Contents

Preface

Everyone wants better health and greater happiness. Despite unprecedented sums spent for health care, the health of most Americans is not getting better. There is concern that many foods commonly eaten do not promote healthy bodies: meat and dairy are too high in fat; too much salt leads to heart problems; highly refined foods lack essential nutrients. Many people worry that conventional medicine, with its emphasis on treating symptoms rather than causes, may not be the best long-term solution. Others want more effective preventive care.

Macrobiotics offers the promise of better health and greater happiness. It is open to anyone who is willing to change their lifestyle and is committed to taking greater responsibility for their health. It is a tool for living within the natural order, helping people eat foods that are suited to their current conditions and the conditions they wish to attain. More specifically, a macrobiotic diet emphasizes whole grains and fresh vegetables, and the proportions are adjusted to meet each individual's needs.

Unfortunately, many people have misconceptions about macrobiotics. It is based on Eastern concepts that may seem alien to people in a Western culture. In addition, many people think that macrobiotics is a bland diet. While people who follow a macrobiotic diet do eat lots of grains and vegetables, no food is absolutely prohibited.

This book seeks to take the mystery out of macrobiotic thinking, and to clarify what a macrobiotic practice can do. It is designed as a reference guide. The first section discusses the various stages of macrobiotics. The second section focuses on foods that are generally eaten by people who are beginning macrobiotics. The third section is an introduction to the principles of macrobiotics and yin and yang, the Eastern concepts that guide food choices. The fourth section presents the macrobiotic view of illness and explains the process of macrobiotic healing.

  May you find here the basis for a long, healthy, and happy life.

What is Macrobiotics?

Macrobiotics is the practical application of the natural laws of change. The term comes from Greek; "macro" means great or long, and "bios" means life. It is a tool that allows one to learn to live within the natural order of life, the constantly changing nature of all things.

Macrobiotics as it is known today is the result of the tireless work and vision of George Ohsawa (1893-1966). Ohsawa developed tuberculosis at the age of fifteen. By the time he was eighteen, his mother, younger brother, and younger sister had all died of the disease. His own illness had progressed to the point that doctors had given up all hope for him. Determined to overcome his condition, Ohsawa began searching for alternative theories of health. He based his theory and practice of macrobiotics on Sagen Ishizuka's (1850-1910) theory of balancing mineral salts, the early heaven's sequence of the I-Ching, yin and yang, and other ancient Eastern concepts. He lived to the age of 73, devoting his life to teaching macrobiotic theory and writing on science, ethics, religion, and philosophy from a macrobiotic point of view.

While macrobiotic principles can be applied to all areas of life, this book emphasizes their application to diet and health. The macrobiotic approach to diet emphasizes whole grains and fresh vegetables. For the most part, it avoids meat, dairy foods, and processed foods. The goal is to provide the body with essential nutrients so that it can function efficiently without loading it with toxins or excesses that must be eliminated or stored. And because the body is always adjusting to changes in the environment and in its own aging process, its needs will always change as well. The idea is to balance the effects of foods eaten with other influences on the body, largely through diet, and to adjust to changes in a controlled and peaceful manner.

A basic tenet of macrobiotic thinking is that all things—our bodies, foods, and everything else—are composed of yin and yang energies. Yin energies are outward moving, yang energies are inward. Every thing has both yin and yang energies, but with either yin or yang in excess. Most of the foods that make up a typical American diet have very strong yin or yang characters and also tend to be acid-forming. In contrast, macrobiotic practice emphasizes the two food groups—grains and vegetables—that have the least pronounced yin and yang qualities, making it easier to achieve a more balanced condition within the natural order of life. Living within the natural order means eating only what is necessary for one's condition and desires, and learning to adjust in a peaceful way to life's changes. Learning the effects of different foods allows one to consciously counteract other influences and maintain a dynamically balanced state. The resulting freedom from fear and the new sense of control are two of the most important benefits of a macrobiotic practice.

A macrobiotic practice encourages the body's natural ability to heal itself. If the body is not burdened by toxins and excesses, it can function better and thus heal any illness that does occur. Anybody who begins a macrobiotic diet goes through a period of healing, beginning with the elimination of accumulated toxins and excesses. Those who are already following a macrobiotic diet may also have periodic health problems and can adjust their diets accordingly. Of course, there are factors other than diet that affect health; true macrobiotic practice emphasizes balancing extremes in all areas. Finally, the goal of macrobiotics is not to avoid death, which is part of the cycle of life. Rather, it seeks to ensure that each person's life is long, healthy, and enjoyable.

The conventional nutritional approach holds that each individual needs certain quantities of proteins, fats, carbohydrates, vitamins, and minerals each day, based on a statistical average of everybody's needs. This makes the recommended daily allowances easy to comprehend but does not allow for the uniqueness of each individual's changing needs. It eventually leads to stagnant thinking. The macrobiotic approach maintains that what works for one person will not necessarily work for another, and that what works one day may not work the next. Therefore, using macrobiotic principles means to determine the foods best suited to you based on your current condition and what you want to become. In other words, a macrobiotic approach requires a change in thinking from a static view of life to a dynamic and flexible one. This leads to real freedom. The first and most important step is to change from a diet based on meat and sugar to one based on grains and vegetables.

Very few people can make such a radical shift overnight. Instead, most people learn macrobiotics in stages.

Beginning Stage

In my experience, the easiest way for relatively healthy people to start a macrobiotic practice is to follow a basic diet that emphasizes whole grains and fresh vegetables. The food we eat affects the way we feel, think, and act. Learning to use macrobiotic principles is much easier after a transitional time of using a basic macrobiotic dietary approach.

The main benefit of a beginning macrobiotic diet is that the body becomes cleaner as toxins and old excesses are discharged. This alone can sometimes relieve minor aches and pains. As our bodies are cleansed, our minds become more clear and our natural good judgment begins to return. People who are in relatively good health may begin a macrobiotic diet after consulting books or relatives or friends who are more familiar with macrobiotic practice. The first section of this book provides all the information that is needed, but a good macrobiotic cookbook is also invaluable.

People with a serious illness should consult a health care advisor or a macrobiotic counselor who is familiar with the effects of dietary change before making big dietary changes. Most people need help learning to use macrobiotic principles effectively to remedy serious illness. A macrobiotic diet must be tailored to the individual's condition. Even two people with the same illness need different dietary adjustments.

Many people who are beginning a macrobiotic diet, or are considering doing so, are taken aback by the number of Japanese foods in a beginning macrobiotic diet. Japanese foods are often emphasized simply because Ohsawa was Japanese. The expression of macrobiotics is becoming less Japanese as more Americans write and teach about macrobiotics.

A second source of confusion is that there are three primary expressions of macrobiotics: that of George and Lima Ohsawa, and those of Ohsawa's students Michio and Aveline Kushi, and those of Herman and Cornellia Aihara. This book unifies their three different expressions of the macrobiotic approach. Still, in consulting any source of macrobiotic information, readers may find seemingly conflicting advice.

Intermediate Stage

In the intermediate stage, one begins to learn the principles of macrobiotics. Macrobiotics is based on the principle that there is a natural order to all of life. What a person does and eats determines who that person is and how that person feels. If one lives and eats in harmony with the natural order, the effect is the natural condition of health and happiness. If one lives and eats in disharmony with the natural order, the result is a condition of minor sickness and, eventually, major sickness. A return to living and eating in harmony with the natural order leads to an improved health condition and outlook on life.

The way to learn about the natural order is to study yin and yang. These Eastern concepts provide a view of life that allows us to live and eat in harmony with the natural order. The knowledge of yin and yang is used to change a weak condition to a strong one, sadness to joy, sickness to health. It is a working knowledge of yin and yang that leads to greater freedom and more control over our health. The second section of this book provides an introduction to yin and yang;

learning how to apply these principles to life is the goal of the intermediate stage. Of course, we can start this stage at any point, even from the first day. As our understanding increases so does our enjoyment of life; as our physical, mental, and emotional health improves so does our judgment. We can better evaluate the appropriateness of advice from others. This increase in confidence leads in general to a more positive outlook toward life.

Advance Stage

At the advanced stage, we have reached the dietary goal of macrobiotics: To be able to eat whatever we want whenever we want without fear. No food is forbidden. This stage is very different from the beginning stage. It is complete freedom rather than a set of rules. Judgment is so developed that we know what to do without having to stop and think about the principles involved. We know the effect of each food and how to counterbalance that effect.

People at the advanced stage realize the importance of sharing their knowledge with others, and they are searching for additional tools with which to better their lives. They understand that macrobiotics does not provide all the answers, but rather is a way of viewing life that can incorporate any and all other disciplines and methods of growth. People at this stage of practice can be recognized by their health, happiness, and honesty.

Benefits of Macrobiotics

In general, the more we know about macrobiotics and the more we practice it, the greater the benefit. However, because every individual is different and no two people have the exact same reaction to changes in diet and lifestyle, the exact benefits for each person differ. Here is a brief list of common benefits:

- ▶ Less or no fatigue.
- ▶ Better health: relief from all pains and sicknesses, including colds, the flu, and cancer.
- ▶ Better appetite, able to eat the simplest food with complete joy and deep gratitude.

▶ Better sexual appetite and more joyful satisfaction.
▶ Deep and good sleep every night without bad dreams.
▶ The ability to fall asleep within minutes of lying down.
▶ Improved memory, leading to better relationships.
▶ Greater freedom from anger, fear, and suffering.
▶ Ability to view difficulties as positive learning experiences.
▶ Better clarity in thinking and promptness in action.
▶ More generosity in our interactions.
▶ Greater control over personal destiny.
▶ The belief that nothing in life is too difficult.
▶ Greater honesty with oneself and others.
▶ Improved understanding of Oneness (God).

Many of these benefits are obviously related to health. In fact, in macrobiotic thought all of these benefits are the product of good health. The third section of this book outlines the macrobiotic view of sickness and healing and provides some information on macrobiotic diagnosis, as well as natural home remedies that can be helpful during the healing process.

The appendix offers guidance for those who have decided to incorporate macrobiotic principles in their lives. Included are:

- ways to start a macrobiotic practice
- a number of exercises for learning to distinguish yin and yang
- using macrobiotic principles
- Ohsawa's order of the universe
- Ohsawa's seven laws and twelve theorems
- Ohsawa's seven stages of judgment

The book concludes with suggested readings and a note on resources.

Macrobiotic Approach to Diet

A Beginning Macrobiotic Diet

The origin of the macrobiotic approach to diet is Ohsawa's relatively complex cosmology called the order of the universe. All life comes from oneness—the infinite, pure expansion. Oneness divides into yin and yang, and from these three all things are created. The inorganic world is created first. This is the world of magnetism, vibration, electricity, atoms, stars, planets, and so on. It is the origin of the organic world. In the organic world, the vegetal world (plants and vegetables) is created first and from it the animal world (animals and humans) is born.

The principal food of humans then should be vegetal foods such as whole grains, fresh vegetables, beans, and sea vegetables. Anything else is a supplement or a luxury. Thus, the macrobiotic dietary approach is to eat a diet largely composed of whole grains and fresh vegetables. This is a major readjustment for people who have been eating a diet based on animal products and canned or frozen vegetables.

Selection

This chapter outlines the foods that make up a basic macrobiotic diet, some of which can be found in supermarkets. However, a local farmers' market or health food store is usually the best source for natural foods, especially for whole grains. Such stores can often offer suggestions for dietary changes, or at least may know of people who follow a macrobiotic approach. Most of the nonperishable foods can be ordered through the mail. (See Resources, page 130, for more information.)

The quality of food is extremely important. No matter what the food, the more natural—the less processed or refined—the better. Try to avoid foods that have been colored; preserved; sprayed with synthetic fertilizers, herbicides, or pesticides; irradiated; or treated in any way with chemicals. Foods grown with genetically engineered seeds should also be avoided. Organically grown or produced foods are preferable; organic foods taste great, reduce health risks, and are best for the health of the soil and water. Select locally grown and seasonal foods as often as possible, especially when buying fresh vegetables. Locally grown foods are most adapted to the local environment, and eating them helps the body to adapt to the local environment as well.

There are an increasing number of convenience foods, such as quick-cooking grains and miso soups, crackers, and snacks. Those without additives, preservatives, or other chemicals are suitable for occasional to moderate use.

Foods

A beginning macrobiotic diet consists of:

grains	40 to 60 percent daily
vegetables	25 to 30 percent daily
beans	5 to 10 percent daily
soups	5 to 10 percent, 1 to 2 cups (bowls) daily
sea vegetables	3 to 5 percent daily
beverages	regularly according to thirst
condiments	several times a week to daily
garnishes/seasonings	small amounts daily, used to balance dishes
pickles	several times a week to daily
fish	0 to 3 times per week

fruit	2 to 3 times per week
desserts	2 to 3 times per week
nuts, seeds, snacks	several times a week to daily
sweeteners	0 to 3 times per week

These food groups are discussed below. Each category contains primary foods (at least 40-50% of the diet) that are used most often in the beginning of macrobiotic practice, secondary foods (at least 25-30% of the diet), occasional foods that are used in small amounts, and foods that should be avoided in the beginning. One should eat a wide variety of foods from each category to ensure a nutritious diet. However, one need not eat all of the foods. People generally base their diet primarily on the foods they like and can find easily.

In the charts that follow, foods are listed in more-or-less yin to yang order. Those foods that should be avoided when you first begin a macrobiotic diet are in italic type.

Note that the recommendations in this section are for those beginning macrobiotic practice. People at the intermediate level who have learned more about yin and yang select foods to suit their condition and surroundings. Those who are more advanced find that they understand the effect of each food and know how to counterbalance that effect.

Finally, people with major illnesses should read the section on Macrobiotic Healing before beginning a macrobiotic diet. Women who are pregnant or breastfeeding should read the chapter on macrobiotic eating for families.

Grains: In temperate climates in the spring and fall, whole grains comprise 40 to 60 percent by volume of daily food consumption. The percentage is increased to 50 to 70 percent in colder climates and seasons, and reduced to 30 to 50 percent in warmer climates and seasons. The grains should be whole and unrefined and may be prepared in a variety of ways.

Of the whole grains, brown rice is the most frequently used, primarily because of its nutritive value and favorable sodium-to-potassium ratio. Of the several varieties, short-grain brown rice is primarily chosen for daily use all year. While any whole grain may be eaten at any time as a primary grain, the heartier ones such as short-grain brown rice, buckwheat, millet, rye, and whole wheat are chosen more in colder climates and seasons, while whole oats, corn, hulled or pot barley, and medium-grain rice are chosen more in warmer climates and seasons. A wide variety of whole grains should be eaten every day.

In practice, many whole grains are consumed in a partially processed form. Examples are cornmeal, rolled oats, bulghur, couscous, creamed cereals, noodles, and flour made from any whole grain. The general recommendation for a beginning macrobiotic approach is to eat mostly whole grains for daily consumption, and to eat products made from whole grains occasionally. Refined or "enriched" grains are avoided in the beginning stages of macrobiotic practice.

Whole and Partially Processed Grains

less yin: ramen noodles, somen noodles, udon noodles, long-grain brown rice, whole wheat crackers, couscous, tortillas, chapatis, cornmeal, corn grits, corn, rolled oats (oatmeal), unsalted rice cakes

less yang: whole oats, pearl barley, wild rice, basmati rice, pot (hulled) barley, buckwheat noodles, medium-grain brown rice, mochi, rye flakes, wheat flakes, sweet brown rice, bulghur, brown rice cream, sourdough whole wheat or rye bread, unyeasted whole wheat or rye bread, rice kayu, cracked rye, lightly salted rice cakes, lightly salted cracked wheat

more yang: rye, whole wheat, quinoa, short-grain brown rice, amaranth, teff, millet, buckwheat

---

Vegetables: Fresh vegetables comprise 25 to 30 percent by volume of daily food consumption. Fresh means vegetables as they come out of the garden—not canned, frozen, or processed in any way. Organically grown vegetables are preferable, the more locally grown the better. Vegetables are prepared in a variety of ways, such as steamed, in a stew or soup, or served raw in salad. Root vegetables are used more in colder climates and seasons, and green leafy vegetables, including raw salads, are used more in warmer climates and seasons, and for balancing heavy meat consumption. A variety of vegetables is eaten daily all year.

In areas with long cold winters, locally grown vegetables, stored without the use of chemicals, are preferable. However, fresh vegetables from another climate are preferred over canned or frozen vegetables. Local farmers in any area should be able to say what foods can be grown and when they are normally available.

Vegetables

extremely yin: *potatoes, eggplant, tomatoes,* shiitake mushrooms, albi, *avocados, sweet potatoes*, mushrooms, *yams, zucchini,* yellow summer squash, patty pan squash, *bell peppers*, artichokes, bamboo shoots, *spinach, Swiss chard,* asparagus, alfalfa sprouts, okra, Jerusalem artichokes, chives, Brussels sprouts

more yin: Chinese cabbage, escarole, kohlrabi, snow peas, green peas, corn on the cob, radishes, string beans, yellow wax beans, purple cabbage, leaf lettuces, endive, cilantro, parsley, bok choy, mustard greens, scallions, collard greens, turnip greens, dandelion greens, beets, broccoli, cauliflower

less yin: kale, green cabbage, celery, butternut squash, buttercup squash, Hubbard squash, acorn squash, Hokkaido pumpkin (kabocha), turban squash, leeks, daikon, onions, watercress

less yang: turnips, rutabaga, salsify, parsnips, carrots, cress, lotus root, burdock

Some macrobiotic teachers suggest that some vegetables should be avoided, or used only occasionally. Eating too much of certain foods can be unhealthy, especially for those with certain health conditions. Many lists of macrobiotic foods are designed to be appropriate for everybody. A better approach—the complete macrobiotic approach—is for each person to learn the effect each food has on his or her body, so that each person can enjoy the widest possible selection of foods nature has to offer.

These are the vegetables that require you to be judicious in using them: the nightshade vegetables, such as potatoes, tomatoes, eggplant, and all peppers other than white and black pepper; those containing large amounts of oxalic acid, such as spinach and beet greens; and other vegetables such as asparagus, avocados, zucchini, sweet potatoes, and yams. They are all extremely yin as shown in the vegetable chart.

Beans, Soups, and Sea Vegetables: Beans, soups, and sea vegetables comprise anywhere from 10 to 25 percent by volume of daily food consumption. Beans are a good protein complement with whole grains, and 5 to 10 percent of the diet consists of bean dishes or soybean products (processed by natural methods without the addition of chemicals) such as miso, natural soy sauce, and tofu used in a variety of ways, including in soups. Soy milk and products made from it are luxury foods used on special occasions, or as transitional foods from a typical American diet to a macrobiotic dietary approach.

A wide variety of soups and stews can be made using any combination of vegetables, grains, beans, sea vegetables, and fish. The most common daily soup in macrobiotic practice is miso soup with vegetables and sea vegetables. Of the many varieties of miso available, barley (mugi) miso is most commonly used daily.

Sea vegetables (seaweeds) grow in and are harvested from the sea. Their nutrient-rich composition and relatively clean growing environment make them an important addition to any vegetal-based diet. They can take time to get used to. Some sea vegetables seem to disappear in bean dishes, and small amounts in soups can be tolerated immediately. Interestingly, sea vegetables are used widely in processed foods, including ice cream, salad dressings, and bread.

Beans and Bean Products

extremely yin: soy milk, bean sprouts, soybeans, black soybeans, split peas, tofu, natto, blackeyed peas, lima beans, whole dried peas, white Northern beans

more yin: tempeh, pinto beans, kidney beans, black beans, black turtle beans, bolita beans, anasazi beans, chickpeas, broad beans, mung beans, red lentils

less yin: aduki beans

more yang: natural soy sauce, miso

Sea Vegetables

less yin: nori, agar agar (kanten), Irish moss, dulse, sea palm, arame, kelp, alaria, nekabu, mekabu

less yang: wakame, kombu, hijiki

Beverages: Beverages are consumed regularly according to thirst and need. Beverages for primary use include bancha twig tea (kukicha), teas made from roasted whole grains such as barley or brown rice, and spring, well, or filtered water. A good source of water is important for maintaining health, especially because most cooking is done with water. Filters that remove chlorine, lead, odors, volatile organic chemicals, and other contaminants from tap water are often a good solution.

Other beverages used in a basic macrobiotic dietary approach are teas and drinks made from vegetables, sea vegetables, grains, beans, or a combination of them. Most macrobiotic cookbooks contain recipes for a wide variety of natural beverages. Fruit juices, soy milk, and naturally fermented alcoholic beverages such as beer, wine, and sake are used for special occasions. Milk and dairy-based drinks, sugared drinks and sodas, coffee, and other stimulant drinks are avoided at first.

While each drink, juice, or tea has its own effect, beverages such as sugared drinks, fruit juices, and herb teas have been grouped for simplicity into their general yin (or yang) category. Some herb teas have a yang effect.

Beverages

extremely yin: *sugared drinks*, natural wine, natural beer, natural sake, fruit juice, soy milk, *coffee*

more yin: green tea, black tea, herb teas, amasake

less yin: carbonated water, mineral water, spring water, well water, carrot juice, vegetable broth, brown rice milk, grain milk (kokkoh), bancha leaf tea

less yang: bancha twig tea, mu tea, kombu tea, dandelion tea, roasted barley tea, roasted brown rice tea

yang: grain coffee (yannoh), ginseng tea, sho-ban tea, lotus root tea, burdock root tea, umeboshi tea

---

Condiments, Seasonings, Oils, and Pickles: Condiments are used as needed to add flavor to cooked dishes and to add nutrients. In addition, they help stimulate appetite and in many cases are an aid to the digestion of grains and vegetables. Gomashio, roasted ground sesame seeds and sea salt, is used for adding salt at the table. The oil from the sesame seeds coats the salt, making the salt easier to process in the body and less yang in effect. Some of the other more popular condiments are listed below. Macrobiotic cookbooks explain how to make or purchase and use these helpful foods.

Seasonings are another way to spice up an otherwise "bland" diet. They are especially helpful to those whose taste buds are adjusting from the highly stimulating typical American fare to a macrobiotic approach. Many seasonings may be used as garnishes for variety in serving or as a complement to help balance the effects of some dishes. For example, grated daikon or grated radish would be a good garnish for fish.

Cooking herbs and spices, including basil, oregano, cinnamon, curry, cloves, and others are used in small amounts. Using natural sea salt is very important because it contains many minerals that are lost during the refining process of commercial salt.

Condiments

more yin: natural mustard (for fish), toasted nori

less yin: powdered sea vegetable, roasted sesame seeds

less yang: ground shiso leaves, gomashio

more yang: scallion miso, tekka, umeboshi plum, shio kombu

Seasonings

more yin: lemon juice, orange juice, brown rice vinegar, umeboshi vinegar, green mustard paste, yellow mustard paste, red pepper, garlic and other herbs

less yin: ground black pepper, grated ginger root, grated daikon, grated radish, grated horseradish

more yang: sauerkraut brine, umeboshi paste, natural soy sauce, miso, umeboshi plums, sea salt

---

Vegetable oils are used in cooking and occasionally for flavoring and in salad dressings.

Pickles are used as condiments. Many macrobiotic advisors recommend eating a small piece of naturally produced pickle after each meal as an aid to digestion. Natural pickles may be purchased at natural food stores or from mail-order suppliers, but many macrobiotic practitioners make their own at home. Avoid pickles made with distilled vinegar.

Oils

extreme yin: coconut oil

more yin: peanut oil, corn oil, olive oil, soybean oil

less yin: canola oil, mustard seed oil, sesame oil, safflower oil

---

Pickles

less yin: pressed salad, sauerkraut

yang: nuka (bran) pickles, takuan pickles, umeboshi pickles

more yang: soy sauce pickles, miso pickles, salt brine pickles, salt pickles

---

Supplemental Foods: Fruit, nuts, seeds, fish, and sweeteners are used as supplemental foods up to two to three times per week within a basic macrobiotic dietary approach. One of the major differences between a macrobiotic diet and other diets is the limited use of fruits, because they contain fructose, a simple carbohydrate that has a similar effect on the body as refined sugar. Still, for a relatively healthy person, eating freshly picked fruit can be one of life's pleasures. Organically grown fruits are preferred, the more locally grown the better. Dried fruits from temperate climates also may be used as part of the weekly amount. Avoid fruits that have been picked unripe or have been sprayed or coated with chemicals before or after picking. Tropical and semi-tropical fruits are avoided on a beginning macrobiotic dietary approach.

Fruit

extreme yin: *mango, papaya, pineapple, bananas, kiwis, dates, figs, grapefruit,* grapes, raisins, green olives, black olives, currants, lemons

more yin: peaches, apricots, plums, prunes, pears, tangerines, nectarines, oranges, honeydew melon, blueberries, watermelon, cantaloupe, mulberries

less yin: apples, cherries, blackberries, strawberries, raspberries

---

Nuts and seeds are used as supplemental foods because they are rich in fat and are somewhat harder to digest than whole grains. In general, smaller seeds and nuts contain less fat and are recommended most. As mentioned earlier, gomashio, a condiment made from sesame seeds and salt, is used daily, or as desired. Nuts and seeds are used primarily as snacks, in baking such as in cakes and cookies, as garnishes, or ground into nut or seed butter.

Nuts and Seeds

extreme yin: Brazil nuts, cashews

more yin: macadamia nuts, pistachios, filberts, hazelnuts, peanuts, pecans

yin: almonds, chestnuts, pine nuts, walnuts, poppy seeds

less yin: squash seeds, pumpkin seeds, sunflower seeds, white sesame seeds, black sesame seeds

---

While the basic macrobiotic diet avoids meat, fish is used as a supplemental food, especially when needed for health; in colder climates and seasons; as extra protein for those active in sports; or as a transition to a grain-and-vegetable-based diet. Less fatty white meat fish is preferable for more regular use, and blue-skinned and red-meat varieties are used for special occasions.

Fish and Seafood

less yang: oysters, bluefish, clams, octopus, tuna, carp, scallops, mussels

yang: lobster, halibut, trout, flounder, mackerel, sole, pike, perch, haddock, cod, swordfish, smelt, scrod

more yang: salmon, shrimp, herring, sardine, red snapper, small dried fish (iriko), caviar

---

Sweeteners are used in desserts and snacks. They are used sparingly (two to three times per week in small amounts) within a basic macrobiotic approach, especially in the beginning. People who are used to a diet high in refined sugar may need to use the listed sweeteners more often as a transition, but none of them replaces the immediate stimulation of refined sugar. (Eventually, naturally sweet vegetables satisfy the need for a sweet taste.) Grain-based sweeteners are preferred. Simple sugars, such as refined sugar, honey, and molasses, are best avoided.

Sweeteners

extreme yin: *mirin*, maple syrup, juice from fruits that grow in temperate climates (such as apples), cooked or dried fruit from a temperate climate

more yin: amasake, barley malt, brown rice syrup

Preparation

Careful and varied food preparation is crucial in a macrobiotic approach. Foods should be tasty and appealing, retain their nutrients, and be appropriate for the people eating them. How a food is cooked changes its quality, and more importantly, its effect on whoever eats it. A more yang food can be made more yin, or a more yin food can be made more yang. One can balance the foods and preparations for a meal so that some are more yin and some more yang, or one can make the entire meal more yin or more yang depending on the season and the needs of whoever will eat the food. A good understanding of food preparation gives the macrobiotic cook flexibility and control over nutrition and health.

The following chart lists some common examples of food preparation methods. In addition, several factors are used to make any of these preparation styles more yin or more yang: the longer the food cooks, and the more pressure, heat, or salt used, the more yang the result; the more water or sweetener and the less time and heat, the more yin.

Food Preparation Methods

more yin: served raw, steaming

less yin: boiling, waterless cooking, sauteing with water

less yang: pressure cooking, sauteing with oil, stir-frying, roasting

more yang: baking, deep-frying, broiling, pressing with salt

extreme yang: pickling, drying

Among the best introductory macrobiotic cookbooks is *Basic Macrobiotic Cooking, Twentieth Anniversary Edition* by Julia Ferré. It provides a straightforward guide to preparing whole grains and fresh vegetables. It and other cookbooks are listed in the Recommended Readings.

Consumption

How food is consumed is important. Chewing food well is most important—the more a food is broken down, the more nutrients will be absorbed by the intestines. Saliva aids in the digestion of complex carbohydrates. People who chew each mouthful fifty to one-hundred times often experience at least a few of these benefits: a reduced tendency to overeat; reduced craving for sweets; reduced desire for excessive amounts of liquid after a meal; better control of salt intake and needs; and greater energy and less overall fatigue.

It is also important to control liquid intake according to thirst and the body's needs. Drinking too much or too little can overwork the heart and the kidneys. Even though grains and vegetables contain a greater percentage of water than animal foods, drinking a sufficient amount of water for proper electrolyte functioning is important.

Quantity also matters. Eating too much food—even good quality, well chosen, properly prepared fare—overburdens the body and can reduce the amount of nutrients the intestines can absorb. Too much of various nutrients can be harmful. For example, too many minerals, such as those from sea vegetables, can cause hardness or tightness in the body. Too much or too little salt can cause fatigue. In general, moderation is one of the keys to a happy and healthy life. One of the benefits of a macrobiotic dietary approach is that it helps people pay attention to what their bodies tell them, making it easy to determine the proper amounts of each food.

How often to eat is an individual decision. But whether one eats two, three, or four times a day, it is best to eat at the same times each day. Proper digestion of foods takes several hours, so eating just before going to bed is not recommended. Some macrobiotic counselors advise not eating for three hours before bedtime. Eating in a peaceful environment also aids in proper digestion and is beneficial to one's health and outlook on life.

Macrobiotic Eating for Families

Because each person is unique and has specific dietary needs, preparing macrobiotic meals for a family may seem very difficult.

However, if everyone in the family is relatively healthy and wants to eat according to macrobiotic principles, it is not difficult to prepare meals that are appropriate for all family members by making a variety of dishes and by using condiments.

Meals for a large family, or for a small family with a great variety of needs, should include at least one dish that is more yang and at least one dish that is more yin. Those who need more yang cooking should simply eat more of the yang dish or dishes and those who need more yin cooking should eat more of the yin dish or dishes. Second, pickles, condiments, or seasonings, which can be used by each family member to adjust the meal to their desire and need, should always be served. Dishes should be prepared keeping in mind the person needing the least amount of salt. Those needing more salt can add gomashio or other salty condiments at the table. At least one dish each day should be high in protein. Those who need more protein can eat a higher proportion of that dish.

If someone in the family is sick or needs to avoid certain foods, there should always be a plain grain dish, such as pressure-cooked brown rice, and a cooked vegetable dish without extensive seasoning. Those who need to avoid certain foods such as sweeteners need to be aware that their condition is temporary and that others in the family may need these foods for their conditions. It is not a good idea to force everyone in the family to eat a restrictive diet because one person is sick.

Macrobiotic cooking in a family where one or more family members refuses to follow a macrobiotic approach is more challenging but still feasible. It is easier if the person who cooks wants to practice macrobiotics. It is possible for other family members to benefit from a macrobiotic approach if the person cooking is willing to prepare dishes at each meal that can be eaten both by those following a macrobiotic approach and those who are not. In practice this means that whole grain and fresh vegetable dishes are available every day. Those following a macrobiotic approach simply avoid the meat, sugar, and other dishes.

Changing to a macrobiotic approach may be difficult for children from the ages of three to sixteen. In general, the older the children the more difficult it can be. Talking openly and honestly is always a good approach; if they refuse, one can still substitute better quality food, such as natural cheese from a natural food store rather than commercial cheese. Gradually introducing more vegetables and whole grain dishes will usually be accepted. If children start to feel better and have more energy and if they see a parent's improvement, they may decide for themselves to adopt macrobiotics. In any case, forcing a diet of grains and vegetables on kids who are used to eating meat and sugar may cause resentment and lead to greater family problems.

Another question that is sure to arise in families with kids is the question of candy. Children aged five and older may require some autonomy. When children are given sugary foods at little league games, scout meetings, friend's houses, or on Halloween, it may be helpful to give them three choices: trade it for a better-quality snack at home, refuse it, or eat it. Refusing is hard. If the children choose to eat the candy, they should pay attention to the effects on their bodies.

A macrobiotic dietary approach is very appropriate during pregnancy and childbirth. If the expecting mother has been following a macrobiotic approach for some time, few adjustments need to be made. Working with a midwife or doctor who has had positive experiences working with macrobiotic families is best. Flexibility is the key to a positive birth experience. Cravings should be satisfied within reason. If a midwife or doctor is concerned about protein, calcium, iron, or any other nutrient, there are many excellent sources of each nutrient within a macrobiotic diet.

If the expecting mother has recently changed to a macrobiotic approach it may be difficult to determine true cravings—something the mother or baby really needs—from cravings for foods the body is still discharging. In this case satisfying the craving is still recommended. If the food that is being craved is filled with chemicals, sugar, or preservatives, determine what the body is really craving, such as the sweet taste, and substitute something of more natural quality.

What should be avoided is profound changes in one's overall

diet during pregnancy and while breastfeeding. The discharge process from an extensive dietary change can be so strong that caution is needed at this time. Major changes in the diet cause discharges of excess toxins; some of these may affect the unborn or breastfeeding baby. Small changes can be made such as finding better quality foods. A complete change from a meat-and-sugar diet to a grain-and-vegetable diet is too drastic during pregnancy or while breastfeeding. Similarly, a major change from a macrobiotic approach to any other dietary approach should be avoided.

The best food for a baby is milk from its mother. The first milk, called colostrum, helps the baby's immune system and encourages the expulsion of meconium wastes that have collected during the time the baby spent in the womb. If for some reason breastfeeding is not possible, there are supplemental drinks that can be made from grains. Consult macrobiotic child care books for recipes, and consult a midwife or health care advisor.

Opinions vary on how long to breastfeed a baby, as well as when and how to introduce solid foods. Like each adult, each baby is unique and has its own needs and desires. Some want and need to breastfeed longer than others. Some want solid food sooner than others. When first introducing solid food, especially before the age of ten or eleven months, the mother should pre-chew the food so that it is mixed with her saliva because babies do not produce ptyalin, an enzyme helpful in the digestion of carbohydrates, before this time.

One concern expressed by doctors and other health professionals is the amount of fat, especially cholesterol, needed by small children for proper brain development. A well-rounded macrobiotic approach along with breastfeeding will supply plenty of the needed fat. However, if breastfeeding is not possible, if the child is developing too slowly, or if there is any other concern over the need for more fat, you should select the most natural quality food possible. Remember, there is no food that is absolutely prohibited in a macrobiotic approach. If dairy foods, meat, or even sugar are necessary for anyone's condition, the macrobiotic approach is to eat that food, buying the most natural product available and eating it only as long as it is necessary. The next chapter discusses the nutritional issues of eating meat, dairy, and other foods.

Nutrients

Each person has different needs. While a macrobiotic diet provides more than adequate amounts of all nutrients, how you feel is a better guide to what you should eat than any list of recommended daily allowances.

The macrobiotic diet contains 12 percent protein, little or none of it from animal sources. It is low in fat (15 percent, including only 2 to 3 percent saturated fat), low in simple carbohydrates (5 percent), and high in complex carbohydrates (68 percent). In contrast, nearly all of the 12 percent of protein in a typical American diet is from animal sources. It is also high in fat (42 percent, including 16 percent saturated fat), high in simple carbohydrates (26 percent) and low in complex carbohydrates (20 percent). (These figures reflect what most Americans eat, not the United States government's dietary guidelines. The diet recommended by the government, like a macrobiotic diet, emphasizes grains and produce.)

The differences between a typical American diet and a macrobiotic diet have important consequences, because what a person eats affects what she or he needs to eat. The body works most efficiently when the proper amounts of nutrients are available, but cannot do its work well when there is too little of a nutrient or when it must work hard to eliminate excesses.

For example, a person who eats a typical American diet high in animal foods and refined carbohydrates needs large amounts of minerals and vitamins such as calcium and vitamin C, very little added salt, and must be careful to get enough dietary fiber. A person who eats foods on a macrobiotic diet needs less calcium and vitamin C, more added salt in cooking, and gets plenty of dietary fiber from whole grains.

The recommended daily allowances (RDAs) are based on the average needs of people who eat a typical American diet. Changes in these daily allowances are based on the needs of those eating large amounts of animal foods. For example, in 1975, the RDAs for calcium and vitamin C were about half what there were in 1995. The recommended daily allowances suggested by the World Health Organization are closer to the needs of people who eat a diet based on grains and vegetables. For example, the United States recommends that a 154-pound male eat 52 grams of protein each day, while the World Health Organization recommends 37 grams. The recommended allowances for a 122-pound female are 44 grams and 29 grams respectively.

Because there is no one macrobiotic diet, it is not possible to perform double-blind studies to show that the macrobiotic diet works. The proof that a macrobiotic dietary approach works for any person is how she or he feels. Furthermore, each person's way of practicing a macrobiotic approach is valid only for that person, because each person is unique. Beware of any studies that show that a specific macrobiotic diet works; the very idea is counter to fundamental macrobiotic principles.

Protein: A majority of people throughout the world eat enough protein with little or no animal food. In fact, a macrobiotic diet contains about 12 percent protein, as does a typical American diet. The only real difference is the source.

Proteins are the building blocks of the body and are used for growth and repair of cells. They are the primary solid constituent of enzymes, hormones, blood, and cellular fluids. Amino acids are the components of protein. After a meal, the body breaks down protein into amino acids, and then reassembles them into the specific proteins it needs. Eight of the twenty-two amino acids are called essential because they can be obtained only from food. These eight amino acids must be eaten at the same meal in certain quantities. If one essential amino acid is lacking, the body can make only a limited amount of usable protein.

Because animal foods contain about the right proportion of all the essential amino acids, they may seem the best source of complete protein. However, they also contain large amounts of saturated fat, which can lead to heart disease and other problems. Also, foods that contain a high percentage of protein, such as animal foods, create many waste products during decomposition that take energy for the body to deal with, and, in excess, overburden the kidneys and liver. Excess protein from animal sources can create toxins from fermentation in the large intestine as well. Complex carbohydrates provide more energy and create less waste products as they are converted to energy, so they are a much better source of energy than animal protein.

A macrobiotic diet approach contains plenty of all the essential amino acids, especially if miso, soy sauce, sesame seeds (gomashio), or beans are eaten daily with whole grains. Grains are high in some essential amino acids and beans are high in others, so when they are eaten at the same meal the body gets all the protein it needs. Nuts, seeds, and fish, which are supplemental foods in a macrobiotic dietary approach, are also good sources of protein. For more about protein and amino acids, see *Basic Macrobiotics* by Herman Aihara, which discusses amino acids and protein requirements at length.

Fat: The body needs fat for a variety of reasons. However, the typical American diet contains about 42 percent fat, and more than one third of this is saturated fat. The health risks of such a diet are well known. Any diet in which fat consumption is more than 20 percent of total intake can lead to problems, including heart disease, cancer, and diabetes.

The macrobiotic diet contains about 13 percent unsaturated fat plus only 2 percent saturated fat. This is enough fat under normal circumstances and is easily obtained from vegetable oils, beans and soy products, whole grains, nuts, seeds, and fish.

Carbohydrates: Because fat provides more than twice as much energy per gram as protein or carbohydrates, many people think it must be the best source of energy. This is not so. First, there are the problems associated with too much fat. Second, animal foods, which are high in fat, are far from natural. They are full of chemicals, additives, hormones, etc. Third, dietary fat converts to body fat much easier than either protein or carbohydrates.

Carbohydrates are a much better source of energy than protein or fat. Complex carbohydrates, such as those in whole grains, beans, and vegetables, are a better source of prolonged energy than the simple carbohydrates in refined grains and processed sugar. Complex carbohydrates take longer to digest and therefore produce a longer-lasting energy supply, whereas simple carbohydrates convert to fat in the body very easily and, in excess, can lead to conditions such as hypoglycemia or diabetes. While a typical American diet contains about 46 percent carbohydrates, over half are simple carbohydrates from refined grains and flour products and simple sugars. A macrobiotic diet contains about 68 percent complex carbohydrates, providing sustained energy over a longer period and producing less waste products than energy produced from protein or fat. Whole grains, vegetables, and beans are excellent sources of complex carbohydrates. Also, these foods are rich in fiber, which ran be very helpful for people with constipation and other problems with the bowels.

Minerals: A macrobiotic diet provides ample minerals. Many people believe that dairy foods, which are rich in calcium, are necessary for a healthy life. Calcium is needed to help build strong bones and teeth. It also helps with blood coagulation, regulates the heartbeat, activates some enzymes, and normalizes the metabolism. A basic macrobiotic diet includes many excellent sources of calcium. Leafy green vegetables such as broccoli, collard greens, kale, and turnip greens are particularly high in calcium. Sea vegetables, soybeans, and soy products also are good sources. Sesame seeds are very high in calcium, making gomashio (ground sesame seeds and salt) an excellent source. Small dried fish (iriko) are a good choice for people who wish to get a large amount of calcium from one source.

Iron is needed by everyone but is of particular concern for women, especially during childbearing years when a significant amount of blood is lost through menstruation and during pregnancy. One of the main functions of iron in the body is carrying oxygen to the

Sources of Minerals

sodium	natural sea salt; miso; sea vegetables, especially dulse; green leafy vegetables; sesame seeds
magnesium	sea vegetables, especially dulse; dried beans, especially soybeans and lentils; leafy greens; whole grains
iron	sea vegetables, especially hijiki; sesame seeds; pumpkin seeds; leafy green vegetables, especially radish tops; millet and other whole grains
iodine	sea vegetables, especially kelp; green leafy vegetables; fish; organically grown vegetables
potassium	sea vegetables, especially dulse and kelp; beans and soy products; vegetables, especially cabbage; nuts; dried fruit
calcium	sesame or other seeds; sea vegetables, especially dulse and hijiki; leafy green vegetables, especially kale and parsley; nuts; soy products
phosphorus	sunflower seeds; beans, especially lentils; grains; sea vegetables

tissues. Iron also activates the formation of bone, brain, and muscle tissue. While a lack of iron is one cause of anemia, magnesium, calcium, copper, vitamin E, vitamin C, many of the B vitamins, and adequate levels of protein are also necessary for building blood. A basic macrobiotic diet includes plenty of sources rich in iron—a 3.5 ounce serving of hijiki (sea vegetable) alone contains almost five times the amount of iron in beef liver. In fact, millet, chickpeas, lentils, soybeans, pumpkin seeds, sesame seeds, and all sea vegetables contain more iron than a comparable amount of beef liver.

Some of the other minerals necessary for a healthy life are sodium, which aids in the formation of digestive juices and helps maintain water balance throughout the body's cells; magnesium, which activates enzymes in carbohydrate metabolism and helps strengthen nerves and muscles; iodine, which stimulates circulation and helps in the oxidation of fats; potassium, which helps regulate the heartbeat and aids in the formation of glycogen from glucose and fats from glycogen; and phosphorus, which helps with the transport of fatty acids, blood coagulation, and the building of strong bones and teeth. Minerals needed in small amounts are known as trace minerals. Sufficient amounts of all these minerals are available within a macrobiotic diet.

Minerals work together. If one is lacking or is too abundant, it affects the proper functioning of all the minerals. This is why it is best not to take megadoses of any one mineral. Any mineral supplement taken should contain a balanced amount of all the major minerals. However, people who eat whole foods and sea vegetables, as in a basic macrobiotic diet, should not need any supplements at all. Natural sea salt is used in a macrobiotic dietary approach because it contains a good supply of trace minerals.

Minerals help produce an alkaline condition in the blood and body fluids so that acidic metabolic by-products can be neutralized. If enough alkaline-forming minerals are not present in the diet, the body uses calcium and any other alkaline-forming minerals it can find, leading to deficiencies and later diseases like osteoporosis. See the chapter on acid and alkaline for more information.

Vitamins: Vitamins are co-enzymes or catalysts. They help the body use the energy in food. Because there are plenty of vitamins in whole foods, people who eat a wide variety of whole grains, fresh vegetables, sea vegetables, and beans do not need vitamin supplements under normal conditions. In fact, synthetic vitamins can be harmful:

Sources of Vitamins

vitamin A   soybeans, carrots, winter squash, rutabagas, other yellow or orange vegetables, broccoli, kale, other green leafy vegetables, nori

vitamin B_1 whole grains, soybeans and other beans, vegetables, seeds, nuts, sea vegetables, especially nori and wakame

vitamin B_2 whole grains, beans and soy products, broccoli, lettuce, cabbage, turnips, sunflower seeds, nori, wakame

vitamin B_3 whole grains, beans and soy products, peas, seeds, nuts, shiitake mushrooms, leafy greens, sea vegetables, especially nori and wakame

vitamin B_6 whole grains, beans, cabbage, nuts

any vitamin supplements should be made from natural sources.

Large amounts of vitamins are not needed by those following a macrobiotic diet. For example, people who eat a lot of animal foods need large quantities of vitamins, including vitamin C, to help break down the protein and use it for energy, especially if the diet is low in complex carbohydrates so that protein is the body's main energy source.

Most food is cooked in a macrobiotic diet. Because cooking destroys some vitamins, some people worry that this approach does not provide sufficient vitamins. The macrobiotic view is that proper cooking minimizes the loss of vitamins and makes the nutrients more accessible to the body by breaking down the tough cellulose walls of the plant cells and that the body has the natural ability to manufacture certain vitamins out of other substances not destroyed in cooking. However, people who have eaten large amounts of animal foods and refined sugar for years can lose this ability, and it may

Sources of Vitamins

vitamin B_{12} sea foods, especially small dried fish (iriko); soy products such as miso, soy sauce, and tempeh; sea vegetables; bacteria bound to the skins of some organically grown vegetables

vitamin C broccoli, parsley, mustard greens, kale, other green leafy vegetables, parsnips, cabbage, carrots, daikon, horseradish, sprouted grains and beans, and fruits, especially strawberries and cantaloupe

vitamin D sunlight

vitamin E whole grains, beans, leafy greens, unrefined vegetable oils, nuts

vitamin K whole grains, radish leaves and other green leafy vegetables, cauliflower, hijiki

take some time of eating primarily grains and vegetables before it returns. If there are no major health concerns that would make raw foods inadvisable, such people should eat more raw foods such as fresh salads, especially in warmer climates and seasons.

Cooking food the proper way, especially over wood or gas heat, condenses the food, making it more yang, without losing the food's vitality. Energy is gained from the heat, from the greater accessibility of nutrients, and from the yangizing of the food. This is not intended to imply that yang is better as both yin and yang foods and preparations are needed for a healthy active life.

Vitamin C (ascorbic acid) receives much attention these days. One of its main functions is helping with protein metabolism, especially in the digestion of animal foods. Because vitamin C cannot be stored in the body, is destroyed by cooking, and is lost with cold, heat, fatigue, and stress, the recommended daily allowance is very high. Macrobiotic thinking is that large quantities of vitamin C are not needed if animal foods are avoided. A more questionable view is that humans should be able to produce their own vitamin C but that they may have lost this natural ability by eating too much of it in the past. In any case, a basic macrobiotic diet includes ample supplies of vitamin C. Good sources of vitamin C in a macrobiotic diet are vegetables, sprouts, pressed salad (with or without salt), and raw salad. Horseradish and daikon are high in vitamin C, which is why they are often served raw (grated) with fish.

All of the vitamins in the B-complex work together. This group includes B_1 (thiamine), B_2 (riboflavin), B_6 (pyridoxine), B_{12}, B_3 (niacin), B_{15}, B_{17}, and biotin, choline, inosital, folic acid, pantothenic acid, paraminobenzoic acid, and Bt (carnitine). These vitamins are the only vitamins that help with carbohydrate metabolism, and they also help with protein and fat metabolism. The bran and germ of whole grains (the outer layers) contain all the B-vitamins needed to metabolize the carbohydrates contained in the whole grains. Refined carbohydrates, such as refined flour and simple sugar, lack the necessary B-vitamins, so that the body uses stored vitamins for metabolism. This results in a net vitamin loss. Vitamin B_1 (thiamine) is one of the most important vitamins. It is destroyed by cooking, especially pressure cooking. However, it can be reassembled in the intestines and can be produced in the large intestines from the cellulose of vegetable foods. Deficiencies in any of the B-vitamins are extremely rare in those following a macrobiotic approach.

A lack of vitamin B_{12} can cause pernicious anemia, a serious disease in bone marrow that inhibits proper blood formation. Vitamin B_{12} is found mostly in animal sources. A study done in Europe, which concluded that macrobiotic children were not getting enough B_{12}, worried many macrobiotic followers, especially those eating no animal products. The non-seafood sources listed above contain small amounts of B_{12}—but then only small amounts are needed. People who think they need more B_{12} should try seafood. If this is not adequate, then a natural supplement may be needed. A more extreme option is injections; once started they may always be needed. Studies have shown acceptable levels of B_{12} in adults who had eaten no animal products at all for more than 17 years.

Vitamin A (retinol and beta-carotene) is in very good supply within a basic macrobiotic diet, and because excessive amounts can be stored in the liver, deficiencies are very rare. A deficiency of vitamin E has never been observed in humans. A deficiency in vitamin K is not likely because healthy people produce vitamin K in the intestines, except immediately after birth or after prolonged treatment with certain drugs.

Vitamin D is made by the cholesterol-related substances in skin when it is irradiated by the sun's ultraviolet rays. Of the more than twenty different forms or analogs of vitamin D, only vitamin D_3, available from sunshine, is natural. Milk is fortified with vitamin D_2, a non-natural analog. Some believe vitamin D_2, actually a steroid, is the root cause of many disorders, and that products containing it should be avoided. Plenty of sunshine, an average of about 15 to 20 minutes of facial exposure per day, is enough for the adequate production of vitamin D. Production is directly related to the surface area of skin exposed to the sun and the darkness of the skin (the lighter the skin the more produced). People who live or work in areas where the sun's ultraviolet rays are obscured much of the time should be careful to spend enough time in the sun when it does shine. If enough time in the sun is not possible, fish liver oil is the only dietary source of natural vitamin D.

In summary, whole foods give whole nourishment. There is no need to worry about the latest findings based on the needs of those who eat a diet based on animal and dairy foods, new drugs, or the newest miracle vitamin or supplement once the body has regained its natural healthy condition.

Acid and Alkaline

The theory of acid and alkaline is a very valuable contribution to macrobiotic thinking. This aspect of proper nutrition is rarely considered within the more conventional approach. It is based on maintaining the proper balance of acid and alkali in the blood. Solutions with a pH of less than 7.0 are acid (the lower the number the greater the acidity), and solutions with a pH of more than 7.0 are alkaline (the higher the number the greater the alkalinity). For a balanced health condition, the pH of the blood should be slightly alkaline—between 7.35 and 7.45—all the time. If the blood pH reaches 6.95 (slightly acid) or 7.8 (slightly more alkaline than normal), death is the result. The pH of the blood is so important that the body has several highly effective blood buffer mechanisms to maintain a constant pH. Thus, many people believe that eating a diet that balances acid and alkaline is not important.

In his book *Acid and Alkaline*, Herman Aihara challenged that view (as well as the idea that acid is always more yin and alkaline is always more yang). Using various scientific methods, Aihara determined which foods are more acid-forming and which are more alkaline-forming once metabolized by the body. The result is four categories of foods: yin acid-forming foods, yin alkaline-forming foods, yang acid-forming foods, and yang alkaline-forming foods.

yin acid-forming foods	yin alkaline-forming foods
grain sweeteners oil nuts beans some grains	beverages fruit sea vegetables seeds most vegetables
most grains fish **yang acid-forming foods**	some root vegetables some sea vegetables salty soy products (miso, soy sauce) sea salt **yang alkaline-forming foods**

Good health depends on eating a balanced amount of acid-forming and alkaline-forming foods (and yin and yang foods) each day. In fact, in my experience most people who have practiced macrobiotics for many years and still feel fatigued much of the time do not pay enough attention to acid and alkaline. They eat too many grains (acid-forming) and not enough vegetables (alkaline-forming), especially raw salads, and not enough sea salt (alkaline-forming).

The situation is more complicated for people who eat a typical American diet. The foods that make up a large part of the American diet, that are not included in a macrobiotic approach, tend to be overly yin and overly acid-forming, making it much more difficult to maintain the body's balance. These foods are also much more extreme both in their yin and yang natures and their acid-forming and alkaline-forming natures than the foods emphasized in a macrobiotic diet. Dairy foods act as buffers. They make acid-forming foods less acid-forming, and alkaline-forming foods less alkaline-forming. However, they do not completely neutralize the effects of strong acid-forming or alkaline-forming foods. Overall, dairy foods tend to be more acid-forming.

Here, then, is a chart of the foods eaten mostly in a modern typical American diet.

yin acid-forming foods most chemicals most medicinal drugs sugar and sugar products psychedelic drugs vinegar and saccharin whiskey and beer most dairy products refined grains	**yin alkaline-forming foods** coffee, honey, and spices fruit raw salads, potatoes
salted cheese poultry red meat and eggs table salt some anti-depression drugs **yang acid-forming foods**	 **yang alkaline-forming foods**

Whether a food is acid- or alkaline-forming is largely determined by its mineral content. The more acid-forming the diet, the more alkaline-forming minerals are needed to metabolize them.

yin acid-forming minerals	yin alkaline-forming minerals
chlorine iodine sulfur phosphorus	potassium iron calcium
	magnesium sodium
yang acid-forming minerals	**yang alkaline-forming minerals**

The typical American diet does not contain enough alkaline-forming elements. Instead, animal foods that produce large amounts of sulfuric and phosphoric acid are consumed. In addition, people are consuming less salt (sodium), an alkaline-forming mineral. While salt in conjunction with large amounts of fat can lead to higher blood pressure and heart problems, the real problem is the fat and not the salt. Because salt is being reduced, the recommended amount of calcium (alkaline-forming) keeps being increased. However, to get enough calcium, people eat dairy products, which produce more sulfuric and phosphoric acid. The cycle continues. The long-term health effects of such a diet are presented in the section on macrobiotic healing.

In contrast, a macrobiotic diet contains foods that break down easily in the body without the need for extra amounts of alkaline-forming elements. In addition, the foods themselves contain alkaline-forming elements in ample supply.

There is one more fact about the balance of acid and alkaline to mention: All active activities such as work, play, worry, and stress cause acid in the body. The opposite and more passive activities such as rest, relaxation, meditation, and breathing deeply help to balance the more active acid-forming activities. An excess of active activities, coupled with a diet of an excessive amount of acid-forming foods, can lead to fatigue and a dulled mental awareness, and then to greater sickness.

Macrobiotic Theory

Macrobiotic principles are the backbone of macrobiotic practice. These principles provide a way of viewing the world that leads to healthful, joyful living. Three of George Ohsawa's main teachings are the order of the universe, the unifying principle of yin and yang, and the stages of judgment. These three teachings equip one with practical tools to use in making daily decisions.

The Order of the Universe

One of George Ohsawa's greatest teachings is his roadmap for understanding the order of the universe, with which one can unleash tremendous power for health and happiness. His spiralic expression of the order of the universe, in which one's origin is traced from Infinity through the universal, inorganic realms to individual, organic life is the heart of Ohsawa's work. Many questions are answered by a full understanding of this framework.

East and West: Ohsawa loved aspects of both East and West and was trying to broker the best of the West to the East and the best of the East to the West. He understood the difference in orientation between the West and the East.

The West, represented by science, starts with what is knowable, visible, or verifiable. This implies that science is limited by the power of its instruments—the telescope or microscope for example. As more powerful ones are made, many scientific "truths" have to be changed. The earth was once thought to be flat with the sun revolving around the earth. The atom was once thought to be indivisible, and so on.

Macrobiotic principles that originated in the Far East begin with that which is unknowable, invisible, and beyond sensory verification. In other words, it starts with the infinite and works toward the finite. This order is unlimited. Science begins with the finite and leaves the infinite out of the equation. Matters beyond the finite are left to religion—a separate field of study that is given little credence in scientific and medical schools. The following paragraph from *Essential Ohsawa* (page 173) summarizes Ohsawa's understanding.

"Both 'visible' and 'invisible' exist, the former measurable in the phenomena of the world we can see, the latter hidden beyond the reach of instruments. The kings of the world of 'visibility' are matter, force, and war, while those of the world of 'invisibility' are spirit, acceptance, and peace. The goal of the world of 'visibility' is relative (satisfaction of desires), while that of the world of 'invisibility' is absolute (awareness of oneness)."

While the West separates matter and spirit, macrobiotic thinking unifies the two. Matter (body) and spirit are not separate from a macrobiotic viewpoint. Understanding this point and changing one's orientation to begin with the infinite rather than the finite is very important in understanding Ohsawa's order of the universe—the basis of macrobiotic theory. Ohsawa organized his order or constitution of the universe into three stages of life and seven worlds.

Oneness: The first stage is infinite, pure expansion that exists beyond the reach of analytical and mechanical measurements. In this world of Infinity or Oneness, there is no separation, and thus no distinguishable thing. It has no beginning or ending and is eternal, transcending both time and space. This infinite, eternal, and absolute world of Oneness is the source of life and of our finite, relative world. In addition, the infinite world continually nourishes the finite world.

Inorganic: Second is the inorganic stage that contains four worlds. This stage occurs whenever and wherever the continuous transcendental expansion divides.

Yin-Yang Polarization: This division creates the world of yin-yang polarization. Other names for yin and yang are outward-moving force or spirals and inward-moving force or spirals, expansive and contractive, and centrifugal and centripetal. The forces of yin and yang are antagonistic and complementary to each other. This polarization is the origin of magnetism—positive and negative charges. The world of yin-yang polarization is created by and is continually nourished by the world of Oneness.

Vibration: The world of vibration begins whenever and wherever the inward yang (+) force and the outward yin (-) force attract and repel each other. This interaction produces waves of light (-), electricity (+), heat (-), chemical energy (+), mechanical energy (-), and gravity (+). Energy produced in this world creates the appearance of space and time, dilation and compression, silence and sound, cold and heat, and darkness and light. The world of vibration is created by and is continually nourished by the worlds of yin-yang polarization and Oneness.

Pre-Atomic Particles: The world of pre-atomic particles occurs whenever and wherever yin and yang combine in variable proportion to produce yin particles and yang particles such as electron (-), neutrino (+), lambda (-), neutron (+), sigma (-), and proton (+). These interactions are controlled by magnetism. The world of pre-atomic particles is created by and continually nourished by the worlds of vibration, yin-yang polarization, and Oneness.

Elements: The world of elements occurs whenever and wherever pre-atomic particles interact with each other due to their polarity to produce atoms and elements such as the noble gases (-), alkali metals (+), the transition metals (-), groups 13 and 14 (+) of the periodic table, groups 15 and 16 (-) of the periodic table, and halogens (+). These interactions are controlled by electricity and are the source of all inorganic substances such as the earth, other planets, stars, galaxies, and solar systems. The world of elements is created by and continually nourished by the worlds of pre-atomic particles, vibration, yin-yang polarization, and Oneness.

Organic: The third stage of life is the organic stage that contains two worlds.

Plants: The world of plants occurs whenever and wherever elements produce fruit (-), flower (+), leaf (-), branch (+), stem (-), and root (+) due to proportional attraction and repulsion of yin and yang and by spontaneous generation. All plants contain chlorophyll, which contains magnesium. The world of plants is created by and continually nourished by the worlds of elements, pre-atomic particles, vibration, yin-yang polarization, and Oneness.

Animals: The world of animals occurs whenever and wherever the magnesium in chlorophyll is replaced by iron. The result is the essence of blood and thus the essence of animals and finally humans. The world of animals is created by and continually nourished by the worlds of plants, elements, pre-atomic particles, vibration, yin-yang polarization, and Oneness. Ohsawa felt that humans are the masterpiece of this creation cycle because humans have the capacity to understand the order of the universe and to live in accordance with its laws.

Seven Laws of the Order of the Universe

In addition to the order of the universe as outlined briefly above, Ohsawa taught seven laws that govern both the Infinite and finite worlds. Here are the seven laws of the order of the universe from the 1962 French edition of *The Atomic Era and the Philosophy of the Far East* as translated by Michael and Maria Chen. Each law is followed by a brief look at how it applies to a particular aspect of life, namely, health and sickness.

Law 1: What has a beginning has an end. The sickness began at some time; it will end at some time. Generally, sicknesses that develop quickly resolve more quickly and those that develop over a longer period of time take longer to resolve. Conversely, health that begins at one time will end at another time.

We "end" our macrobiotic practice every time we change it. We, then, begin with a new understanding. In this way, we have a daily macrobiotic practice that "begins" anew with each sunrise. We have a weekly, monthly, seasonal, and yearly macrobiotic practice, each "ending" and "beginning" with each new week, month, season, and year.

We can begin anew at any moment, realizing that it will, and must, "end" at some other moment. We don't need to hold on to what we begin. We can let go. This is freedom. We can let go of our macrobiotic diet, our brown rice, our ego attachments. We need not fear the "end" because every moment is a new beginning. We can accept everything with great pleasure and thanks.

Law 2: What has a front has a back. If health is considered the "front," then sickness is the "back." This statement is not judgmental; however, most of us see the front (in this case health) as good and the back (in this case sickness) as bad. A more complete understanding sees both as necessary.

If we learn to accept everything, then we can accept sickness with the same sense of gratitude as we accept health. This is usually not the case however. We don't accept sickness like health, misfortune like happiness, war like peace, poverty like prosperity, enemy like friend, or death like life. We are human. We want health, happiness, peace, prosperity, friends, and life—not their opposites.

We tend to view sickness as a punishment rather than as an opportunity. Sicknesses show us that we are violating the order of the universe. We have only to learn in what way and to adjust our actions accordingly.

Combining the first two laws, we can see that any sickness is temporary. Curing any temporary sickness leads only to temporary health. Learning how to remedy unwanted conditions is valuable and worth our efforts. However, unless we see the bigger picture, our understanding remains stuck in the world of opposites. True happiness comes from being able to embrace both halves of any pair of perceived opposites with unconditional gratitude.

Law 3: There is nothing identical. Everyone's personal condition is different and constantly changing. The trick is to learn how to turn one's condition in the desired direction. What works for one person isn't necessarily the right solution for another. Each person's attitude, living conditions, lifestyle, and diet are not only unique to that person, but also must be adjusted daily depending on various factors.

The prescriptive, standard macrobiotic diet is very valuable, but it is an introductory diet only to be followed for a short period of time. Once the principles are studied and understood, one moves on to making daily choices based on the principles rather than following a prescriptive approach.

Understanding that there are many ways to practice macrobiotics is most important. All have value. There is nothing identical. Thus, true macrobiotics is unlimited. If we can learn to spend more time accepting, and less time judging others and ourselves, we can take a big turn toward real health, the unification of temporary sickness and health.

Law 4. The bigger the front, the bigger the back. This law means, the greater the health, the greater the potential sickness, and conversely, the greater the sickness, the greater the potential health. The greater the difficulty (sickness), the greater the joy (health).

Nuclear energy is a clear example of something with a big front and a big back—it can be of great benefit in filling growing energy demands. On the other hand, all it takes is one nuclear accident to remind us of one of the potential dangers. Its use as a weapon is another. Conflicts between nations are made more tense by the proliferation of nuclear weapons.

Macrobiotics can be of great benefit. A brief list of common benefits of macrobiotic practice may be found on pages 11-12. This fourth law reminds us that macrobiotics can also lead to the opposite, great harm or sickness. The greatest sickness is arrogance— the thinking that we are better than others, smarter than others, and healthier than others because of our diet and lifestyle. We need to guard against such thinking and to unify all apparent opposites.

Law 5: Every antagonism is complementary. A perceived sickness is seen as antagonistic to us. Yet, the sickness also is complementary—a necessary part to complete the whole. We know what it means to be healthy because we know what it means to be sick. Both are necessary.

There is a lesson to be learned in each thing that happens to us. If we do not learn the lesson, we are bound to repeat it. Everything that we view as antagonistic and unbearable (sickness, poverty, war, and so on) is also complementary. It happens to us because it is what we are lacking. We need to embrace these antagonisms. Destroying them is not the answer. While we might temporarily succeed in doing so, it only comes back in a stronger form. Once we learn to view everything that happens to us as a benefit, we become closer to overcoming the fear of getting sick and to truly curing any disorder.

Law 6: Yin and yang are the classifications of all polarization. They are antagonistic and complementary. Rewritten with sickness and health substituted for yin and yang we have: Sickness and health are the classifications of every person's condition. They are antagonistic and complementary. Again, both are necessary. Sicknesses provide us with the opportunity to learn, to grow, and to elevate our judgment.

Here with the sixth law, Ohsawa reiterates the fact that every antagonism, including yin and yang, is complementary. There is a tendency among macrobiotic practitioners to believe that yang is good and yin is bad. This is simply not the case. Both are necessary. It is the unification of the two that is important. Likewise, we see health as good and sickness as bad. Once we can see that both are necessary and that the unification of the two is more important, we are on our way to understanding health and sickness in a more complete way.

Law 7: Yin and yang are the two arms of One (Infinite). Both health and sickness are part of One Infinite. The Infinite accepts both and so should we. Truly understanding these last two laws can lead to the remedy of any unwanted condition.

Summary

Here is the essence of macrobiotic understanding. We all come from One Infinite. We are all part of One Infinite, and always will be. We have reached unification—the world of no separation. Yet, we were born into this world of opposites with temporary sickness and temporary health, with things we like and things we don't.

Starting with duality, the world of opposites, it is difficult to comprehend One Infinite. It is like trying to put Humpty Dumpty back together again. If we view things from the perspective of One Infinite, however, we begin to appreciate that everything that happens to us is for our benefit. We have only to humbly accept and to give thanks.

Some may argue that accepting everything means resignation, giving up. It does not. If we truly accept everything, we accept our humanity. We accept our desire to change things to their opposites. We accept those things we dislike. We accept our arrogance. We accept everyone else for each person's journey is unique. We accept every challenge and each moment of Grace with equal joy.

If we can do all these things, then we begin to see things in a different way. We are ready to begin a macrobiotic practice with a new set of eyes—with the magic spectacles Ohsawa gave us to help increase our understanding. We are ready to begin anew, fully accepting all that comes our way on life's wondrous journey.

Unique Principle

The unique principle is George Ohsawa's interpretation of the Far Eastern concepts of yin and yang and how to use them in our daily lives. Because his idea is to learn how to unify all apparent opposites, Ohsawa also used the term unifying principle in much of his writings. Both terms are used in this book.

Macrobiotic Yin and Yang

At the root of macrobiotic thinking is the realization that there is a natural order to life: day turns to night and night to day; spring follows winter, followed by summer, autumn, and winter again; inhaling is followed by exhaling, the heart expands and contracts in the pumping of blood throughout the body. These changes take place whether or not we pay attention to them.

The words "yin" and "yang" help classify and categorize things within this natural order. They have meaning only when used to describe or compare things. Yang represents the inward or contracting force of life, and yin represents the outward or expanding force. The first step in learning to use yin and yang is to learn how to classify things as either more yin or more yang.

In terms of space, when the heart is expanding it is becoming more yin. When the heart is contracting it is becoming more yang. Similarly, when the lungs are expanding while inhaling they are becoming more yin, and when the lungs are contracting during exhaling they are becoming more yang. Yin always follows yang and yang always follows yin, in the same way we breathe in and then out. This is the natural order of all things.

Macrobiotic practice is to study and then intentionally live within this natural order. There is always change from yin to yang and yang to yin. The macrobiotic idea is to have calm change instead of violent change, orderly change instead of chaotic change, comfortable and healthy change instead of unpleasant change involving sickness. In fact, people begin to return to the natural order once they begin to eat more natural foods and less processed and chemicalized foods. The ability to comprehend yin and yang increases the more natural foods they eat and the more they study.

Any pair of opposites can be classified as more yin or more yang. Some of these classifications make sense immediately, while others require more thought.

Charting opposites is relatively easy because the difference between yin and yang characteristics is very great. For example, it is

more yang	more yin
contractive	expansive
inward	outward
fire	water
hot	cold
heaviness	lightness
inner	outer
active	passive
drier	wetter
summer	winter
day	night
brighter	darker
descending	ascending
time	space

easy to say that 30 degrees Fahrenheit is cold and therefore more yin. Similarly, 100 degrees is hot and therefore more yang. But what about 65 degrees? Is it more yin or more yang? Compared to 30 degrees 65 degrees is warmer, and therefore more yang. Compared to 100 degrees, however, 65 degrees is cooler, and therefore more yin. This is nothing more than what one instinctively knows. If one is cold (more yin), she or he seeks warmth (more yang). If one is too hot (more yang), she or he seeks coolness (more yin). To put it another way, the natural order is to unify all opposites. Somebody who is too yin or too yang seeks the opposite quality in order to become more centered, calm, orderly, comfortable, or healthy.

Note that the macrobiotic usage of yin and yang is different from the way yin and yang are used in Chinese or Oriental Medicine. Chinese Medicine uses yin and yang as a curative technique. The macrobiotic way uses yin and yang as a way to restore natural order and gain freedom. Both systems work, and many macrobiotic followers and counselors have learned both usages in order to understand life more fully.

The Twelve Theorems of Yin and Yang

George Ohsawa wrote volumes on the natural order of the universe and yin and yang, which he called "the twelve theorems of the unique principle." Here are the twelve theorems as written by Ohsawa in the 1962 French edition of *The Atomic Era and the Philosophy of the Far East* as translated by Michael and Maria Chen. Following each theorem, I have reworded and expanded on these principles, especially as related to health and sickness. Of course, there is much more to say about each one, and many more principles for further study (see the Recommended Readings, page 126).

1. Yin-Yang are two poles which enter into play when the infinite expansion manifests itself at the point of bifurcation.

Yin and yang come from Oneness, the Infinite, and represent the two fundamental forces (outward and inward) or activities of Oneness. For any thing or phenomenon to exist in this finite world, its opposite must also exist. For example, we know what it is to feel well only because we know sickness. Both health and sickness are manifestations of the Infinite.

2. Yin-Yang are produced continually by the transcendental expansion.

Yin and yang are produced infinitely and continuously from Oneness. Health and sickness are produced continually by the transcendental expansion, which is beyond our experience but not beyond our intuitive knowledge. Developing this intuitive knowledge, or listening to one's intuitive voice, is most important.

3. Yin is centrifugal. Yang is centripetal. Yin and Yang produce energy.

Yin activity is the outward, centrifugal force and produces expansion, lightness, cold, and so on. Yang activity is the inward, centrifugal force and produces contraction, heaviness, heat, and so on. Sickness is centrifugal (moving or directed outward from the center). Health is centripetal (moving or directed inward toward the center). Health and sickness produce energy. Without one or the other, there is no energy and thus no life.

4. Yin attracts Yang. Yang attracts Yin.

Everything is attracted to its opposite. Someone who is more yin will be attracted to people and things that are more yang, and vice versa. The finite world only exists as long as opposites exist. Sickness attracts health. Health attracts sickness. By unifying opposites one reaches toward the infinite world of Oneness where there is no separation, and thus no opposites. The ability to unify opposites is one key to a happy and healthy life.

5. Yin and Yang combined in variable proportion produce all phenomena.

An infinite variety of combinations and proportions of yin and yang produces energy and all other things, both visible and invisible. Without the fundamental forces of opposition (yin and yang), nothing, including life, would be possible. Health and sickness combined in variable proportion comprise all persons' individual conditions. There is a force of attraction toward health and repulsion from sickness in every person's condition. We try to avoid sickness. We try to maintain health.

6. All phenomena are ephemeral, being of infinitely complex constitutions and constantly changing Yin and Yang components. Everything is without rest.

Every thing is constantly changing its yin and yang characteristics—every thing is restless. What is more yin one day can become more yang the next, and vice versa. In my experience this is the hardest principle to understand, but it is also the most rewarding. It allows one to change an overly yin condition of sickness to a more healthy balanced condition. Health becomes sickness and sickness becomes health. The real question is the direction one's condition is heading. It is this theorem that Ohsawa used to state that all sickness could be "cured" in ten days. Because the quality of one's blood can change in ten days, Ohsawa reasoned that the direction could be changed from sickness toward health in that period of time.

7. Nothing is totally Yin or totally Yang, even in the most apparently simple phenomenon. Everything contains a polarity at every stage of its composition.

Every thing in this finite world is composed of both yin characteristics and yang characteristics. There is nothing that is all yin or all yang. In other words, yin and yang are not absolute qualities; they are relative qualities. This is one of the most important principles of yin and yang theory. No one is totally well or totally sick, even in the most apparently simple case. Every condition contains a polarity at all times. There will be sickness of varying degrees in times of health and varying degrees of health in any instance of sickness. Realizing this can lead to less worry when sicknesses become more noticeable.

8. Nothing is neutral. Yin or Yang is in excess in every case.

There is nothing that is neutral. Either yin or yang is in excess at any given time within every thing. If the yin characteristics dominate, then the thing is called "more yin." If the yang characteristics dominate, then the thing is called "more yang." If the yin or yang characteristics dominate, but just by a little, then the thing is called "less yin" or "less yang." Health or sickness is in excess in every case. We perceive ourselves as healthy or sick at every moment, even though at any moment a healthy condition can turn toward sickness or a sickness can turn toward health.

9. The force of attraction is proportional to the difference of the Yin and Yang components.

The force of attraction between two things is directly proportional to the difference of yin and yang in them. For example, something that is extremely yin and something that is extremely yang will have a much greater affinity than something that is extremely yin and something that is less yin. The force of attraction is proportional to the difference of the health and sickness components. The greater the perceived sickness, the more attention we give to that sickness.

10. Yin repels Yin and Yang repels Yang. The repulsion is inversely proportional to the difference of the Yin and Yang forces.

The more alike two things are, the more they will repel each other. The farther away or less alike they are, the weaker the repulsion. Someone who is more yang will be repelled by people and things that are more yang, and vice versa. Sickness repels sickness and health repels health. The force of repulsion or attraction is inversely proportional to the degree of health or sickness. When we perceive ourselves in good health, there is more opportunity and likelihood for us to become more complacent or uncontrolled, leading toward the direction of sickness.

11. With time and space, Yin produces Yang, and Yang produces Yin.

At the extremity of development, yin becomes yang and yang becomes yin. In other words, over time, and within the space of the finite world, health produces sickness, and sickness produces health. Every person's condition will change sooner or later as long as we live. Because many of the charts in macrobiotic literature are two dimensional, people see yin and yang as opposites. But, if one thinks of the seasons, it is easier to see how more yin (winter) can become more yang (summer), and vice versa.

12. Every physical body is Yang at its center and Yin toward surface.

The surface (periphery) of every thing is more yin and the center of the same thing is more yang, because yin is the representation of the outward force and yang is the representation of the inward force. Every physical body is healthier at its center and sicker toward its surface. The body's highest priority is to protect the vital internal organs. The signals of sickness manifest or show first on the surface of the skin and on our hands and feet (the extremities). Learning how to read these signals or symptoms of sickness can be invaluable.

While everything in this finite world has yin and yang aspects, macrobiotic practice emphasizes the yin and yang of food and of the body. What one eats influences what one thinks and as such is an important determinant of health.

Yin and Yang of Food

Macrobiotic teachers have determined how yin or yang various foods are from theoretical understanding, practical experience, or a combination of both. All foods have many yin and yang qualities. These are some of the aspects of each food that must be considered:

Yin and Yang Qualities of Food	
Composition	
more yang	**more yin**
rich in sodium	rich in potassium
more dry (less watery)	more watery (less dry)
high in complex carbohydrates	high in fat
Color and taste	
more yang	**more yin**
red, brown, orange, yellow	white, green, blue, violet
darker shades of color	lighter shades of color
bitter, salty	sweet, sour, spicy
Growth	
more yang	**more yin**
downward or inward force	upward or outward force
vertical below ground	vertical above ground
horizontal above ground	horizontal below ground
slower growth	faster growth

Season and Climate in the Northern Hemisphere

more yang	more yin
grown more in winter months	grown more in summer months
grown in colder climates	grown in warmer climates
(grows bigger or more abundantly in the North)	(grows bigger or more abundantly in the South)

Manner of production or processing

more yang	more yin
organically grown	grown with chemical fertilizers
needs longer cooking time	needs shorter cooking time
whole food	refined food

Size, weight, and hardness

more yang	more yin
smaller, shorter	bigger, taller
heavier, harder	lighter, softer

To determine the placement of each food on a chart, all the factors or characteristics are taken into consideration. However, it is not an exact science. Adding up all the yin and yang characteristics of any food is very subjective. First, just how much more yin or more yang each food is for each aspect must be determined. Then, how much weight to give each aspect must be calculated in order to reach a sum total.

In practice, after the measurable theoretical considerations are noted, a final decision is made based on the observable effect of each food. Because every person is different and reacts differently to various foods, these decisions are somewhat subjective. Since the first yin-yang charts of foods were made by George Ohsawa, newer charts have been made that reflect the theoretical understanding and practical experience of more recent writers. In fact, different books list foods in slightly different yin to yang orders. All macrobiotic food charts are most useful as general guidelines. Ideally, everybody should create their own charts, based on how foods affect them.

Here is a detailed list of food categories from more yang to more yin.

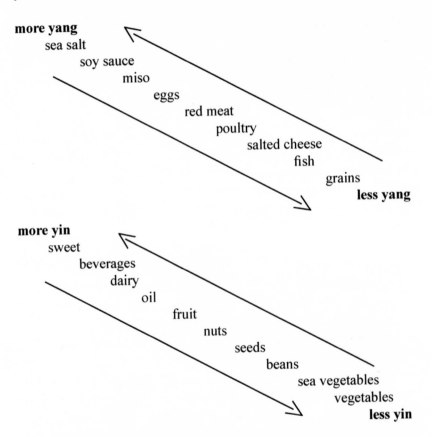

The yin or yang qualities of foods within one category may overlap the yin or yang qualities of foods in other categories. For example, an extremely yin vegetable such as a potato is more yin than a less yang sea vegetable such as kombu, even though sea vegetables as a category are more yin than vegetables.

This leads to some confusing terminology in the macrobiotic literature. For example, in the macrobiotic literature bananas are said to be more yin and strawberries are said to be more yang. But in fact, strawberries produce a yin effect and not a yang effect because the whole category of fruits is more yin. This is confusing. Therefore, the charts in this book more clearly reflect the actual yin and yang qualities of foods. The terms "extreme yin" and "extreme yang" and "less yin" and "less yang" are used to further differentiate among the various yin and yang qualities.

The food and preparation charts in the beginning macrobiotic diet chapter along with the understanding gained in this chapter may be used in deciding what to eat each day. They may be used to prepare balanced meals or to tilt the meal toward yin in the summer or toward yang in the winter. They may also be used to correct an overly yin or yang condition by preparing meals emphasizing the opposite quality. Because the principal foods used in a macrobiotic diet are those with the least pronounced yin or yang qualities and are more toward the center than those in a typical American diet, one can prepare healthy balanced meals with relative ease.

Yin and Yang of the Body

The condition of the body is continually changing as it reacts to foods eaten, the seasons, aging, situations in one's life, and all other aspects of one's daily environment. Macrobiotic practice emphasizes the role of food in both determining a person's condition, and changing it. A person's overall condition is determined by many different factors, such as whether the pulse is weak or strong, the person is more extroverted or introverted, thinks more about the past or the future, or prefers physical activities to mental activities. Some of these conditions, such as height, do not change much. Others, especially emotional conditions, can change in a moment. A mix of yin and yang conditions is needed for a balanced, healthy life. However, if any factor, or group of factors, becomes extreme enough to cause discomfort, this can lead to trouble, signaling a need to move that factor, or group of factors, toward the center area.

Every thing always seeks its opposite. If extreme yin foods such as sugary foods are eaten, the body becomes more yin. Seeking the opposite quality, the body craves meat or salt (more yang). Eating an excess of meat or salt, the body becomes more yang and seeks yin again. Furthermore, the body is never completely balanced—yin or yang is always in excess. The natural order is yin and yang changing into each other, forever. The goal of macrobiotic practice is to make the changes in a more comfortable way within a comfortable range of dynamic balance.

Yin and Yang of the Body	
Physical condition	
more yang	**more yin**
strong pulse	weak pulse
red face, pink face	yellow face, pale face
drier (less watery)	(less dry) wetter
smaller, shorter	bigger, taller
heavier, harder, stronger	lighter, softer, weaker
Emotional condition	
more yang	**more yin**
laughing, over joyous	sadness, crying
anger, complaining	worry, whining
overconfidence, arrogance	inferiority, doubt or fear
stubborn, screaming	complacency, silence
Psychological condition	
more yang	**more yin**
extrovert, aggressive	passive, introvert
optimist, positive thinker	negative thinker, pessimist
focused	spaciness
talker	listener

Mental condition	
more yang	**more yin**
specific thinker	universal thinker
dealing with the past	dealing with the future
materialistic	spiritual
Activity	
more yang	**more yin**
physical, social	mental, emotional
jogging, dancing	meditative, sleeping
disco, rock and roll music	blues, religious music
talking	writing

I have not placed male and female on the list, as macrobiotic literature does, because it leads to the wrong conclusion that females are, or should be, more yin and males are, or should be, more yang. Every person has both yin and yang characteristics and should determine the proper combination for their condition and desires. One can change an overly yin or an overly yang condition to a more balanced and healthy condition. First, one pays attention to the body's condition and how it changes each day. If any particular quality becomes overly yang or yin, and causes discomfort or gets one in trouble, one does the opposite to move oneself back to a more balanced condition. Someone who is too yang should eat more yin foods and engage in more yin activities. Someone who is too yin should eat more yang foods and engage in more yang activities. For example, someone who drives to work gripping the steering wheel tightly and getting angry at other drivers needs to loosen up (become more yin). Someone who does not pay attention to how her or his driving is affecting others' needs to become more focused (more yang).

Ohsawa suggested checking one's daily eliminations. An overly yang condition of the stools implies that more yang food was consumed. Less salt and a greater proportion of yin foods would be the remedy. An overly yin condition implies that more yin food was consumed. More salt or a greater proportion of yang foods is suggested. Dark urination usually indicates an excess of salt (sodium) and light or clear urination often means too much liquid was consumed. The general guideline is for males to urinate three or four times in twenty-four hours, and for females to urinate two or three times per day. It is normal for those over fifty to urinate more often.

Yin and Yang of Daily Eliminations	
Stools	
more yang	**more yin**
darker in color	lighter or greenish in color
harder, constipated	softer, diarrhea
Urination	
more yang	**more yin**
darker in color	lighter in color
less frequent	more frequent

Many disorders can have both a yin cause or a yang cause as will be explained in the next chapter. The overall idea of macrobiotic diagnosis is that the part reflects the whole, so that any part gives a picture of the whole condition. For example, each part of the face corresponds to a different organ. Every aspect of the body can be more yin or more yang, and books on diagnosis study everything from the top of the head to the bottom of the foot, including voice, body odor, and conditions such as stiffness. Here are just a few examples of very specific indicators.

Some Specific Yin and Yang Indicators	
Eyes	
more yang	**more yin**

eyeball low
   (white showing above)
	eyeball high
	   (white showing below)

narrow distance apart	wide distance apart

smaller or slanting
   downward
	larger or slanting
	   upward

iris turned inward
   (toward the nose)
	iris turned outward
	   (toward the ears)

Nails	
more yang	**more yin**
convex, downward at end	concave, upward at end
short, wide	long, narrow
Shoe Wear	
more yang	**more yin**
front wears out first	heel wears out first
more wear on the inside	more wear on the outside
Baldness	
more yang	**more yin**
back of head	front of head, top of head

Stages of Judgment

The seven stages or levels of judgment are Ohsawa's theory of how consciousness develops. There are six stages of relative consciousness to Universal Consciousness (the seventh). These stages describe our spiritual growth from the moment of conception (individual life) until our return to Infinity or Oneness.

First Judgment: Physical or Mechanical

Physical judgment begins almost immediately after birth. Instinct or unconscious reflexes guide our actions. When we are hungry, we cry. When we are thirsty, we cry. When we feel a sense of separation, we cry. Someone comes to our aid.

Physical judgment leads to the tendency to be habitual. We form habits, some of which are helpful. It seems to be easier to do the same things or to eat the same foods every day. If and when habits become entrenched to the point that a change in thinking or action is impossible, such habitual thinking becomes harmful to our adaptability.

For Ohsawa, blind, mechanical, physical judgment is most important because without it we cannot live. Bacteria and microbes attack the body constantly. The body's defense mechanisms automatically destroy them. This is physical judgment. Without it we cannot live. We have physical judgment throughout our individual lives. Our work is to strengthen it and to keep it strong. Here are some ideas to enhance physical judgment:

- Be creative daily in expressing yourself by writing, singing, dancing, cooking, painting, drawing, acting, and so on, or in thinking of ways to help others.
- Engage in healthy practices such as chewing food well and concentrating on breathing deeply and completely.
- Have more contact with Nature by spending as much time as possible in the cleanest environment you can find.
- Create movement anywhere there is stagnation by beginning an exercise program appropriate for your condition or through a change in dietary approach.
- Initiate flexibility anywhere there is rigidity by reacting to new ideas with openness and to difficulties as beneficial challenges.

These activities help us become more adaptive, leading to real health. Real health contains periods of temporary sickness and temporary health. Our efforts in strengthening physical judgment can be invaluable on our temporary journey between birth and death.

Second Judgment: Sensorial

Our sensorial judgment begins some days after birth. This judgment develops into the ability to distinguish colors, sounds, smells, tastes, and textures. We begin to sense the difference between what is agreeable and disagreeable.

Sensory judgment leads to the desire for comfort and enjoyment in life. When we were babies, our parents did everything they could to make us comfortable. When our parents become older, we have the chance to reciprocate. We allow them to move into our homes. We place them in nursing homes when they need more care than we can provide. We ask physicians to make them as comfortable as possible during hospital stays and procedures. Every decision we make is with their comfort, and with our comfort, in mind.

Our desire for comfort and enjoyment begins very early in life and continues throughout our days. We can deepen our enjoyment of life through nourishment of our senses, leading to greater sensitivity. Here are some ideas to strengthen sensorial judgment:

- Consume foods in as unaltered a form as possible, avoiding chemicalized foods and those with artificial additives or preservatives.
- Recognize the importance of finding good-quality air to breathe, sunshine to absorb, water to drink, clothes to wear, and cosmetics to use.
- Broaden the definition of food to anything taken into body, mind, or Spirit.
- Realize we also are nourished by what we read, see, hear, touch, feel, and smell – the books we read, the music we listen to, the television programs we watch, and even the people we associate with may greatly affect our well being.
- Nurture yourself by giving to others, recalling Ohsawa's instruction to give, give, give, infinitely.

These activities help us become more sensitive, leading toward complete happiness. Complete happiness includes times of joy and laughter and periods of sadness and tears. There is no immunity from difficult times. We all experience pain and suffering during our lifetimes. By increasing our sensitivity, we can nurture ourselves and others during these times regardless of the particular circumstances.

Third Judgment: Sentimental or Emotional

Sentimental or emotional judgment begins some months after birth. This judgment develops into the ability to discriminate. We begin to discern what we like versus what we dislike. This stage of judgment should not be dismissed. Development of sentiment is of vital importance to our growth as human beings.

When we receive criticism, our initial response is usually emotional because we dislike being criticized. We become upset. Our emotions become unstable. Stabilizing emotions can take time and requires patience. Waiting at least 24 hours and then rereading criticism in as realistic a way as possible will yield a more balanced response, or at least a less combative one.

While it would take an entire book to adequately cover this subject, learning to express feelings is of primary importance. Burying emotional responses leads away from health. Becoming more capable of conveying emotions in an effective way leads us in a positive direction and toward greater emotional stability.

Physically we grow throughout our younger years. By developing our sentimental/emotional judgment, we grow in mind and Spirit. Such growth allows us to realize more of our potential and to develop greater stability and expressiveness. Here are some ideas to develop sentimental judgment.

- Eat as great a variety of foods as your condition allows.
- Explore new ideas from as great a variety of sources as possible.
- Realize that the tendency of everything in life is to increase—avoid blocking growth by not burying emotions or other means.

- Live with a sense of gratitude and thankfulness according to the biological law: from one grain comes ten thousand.
- Recognize that while physical growth is limited, spiritual growth is unlimited.

These activities help us become more emotionally stable. By growing or increasing our patience and expressiveness, we become more peaceful, leading toward the realization of eternal peace.

Fourth Judgment: Intellectual

We begin to ask questions around the age of 4. We want to know how things work. We drive our parents crazy all the time by asking, "Why?" This is intellectual judgment—the development of an interest in gathering knowledge.

Intellectual judgment leads to the desire to be correct or accurate. We want to choose the right foods and to prepare and consume then in the proper way. However, acquiring knowledge can be a trap. We can increase our knowledge until we block learning by thinking we know everything all already.

We tend to view knowledge in a finite way. Our opinion is: The more we know, the less there is that we don't know. However, everything in life increases, including the amount of knowledge. The more we know, the more there is that we don't know. When we truly comprehend this, we are humbled. We can accumulate all the knowledge our mind allows, but we must be aware that there is always more. Here are some ideas to increase intellectual judgment.

- Realize that quantity affects quality—too much "good" food is no better than a small amount of "bad" food just as too much knowledge can be harmful when it blocks us from accepting new ideas or from seeing our true nature.
- Learn from mistakes, books, Nature, others, and yourself—everything in life is for our benefit.
- Question everything and answer your own questions— find out for yourself rather than blindly believing others.

- Be totally honest with yourself and others.
- Accumulate without arrogance.
- Realize that the primitive is as likely to understand the true meaning of life as the most educated person.

These activities help us experience life in a more complete way. We become aware of our place in life as we gain insight and wisdom. This can lead us toward illumination and enlightenment—clarity of our connection to universal consciousness.

Fifth Judgment: Social

Social judgment develops out of the desire to have companionship with others. Around the age of six, we want to be the same as others. We want to have friends. Later, in our teen years, we desire to be different from others. We begin to seek and to express our uniqueness and independence.

Social judgment leads us to our expressions of morality. We begin to recognize that our actions affect the common welfare. We can live with others in harmony or discord. We can accept our responsibilities and live in a way that is considerate of others. Or, we can deny any such mandate and think only of ourselves. We, and the nations we live in, can take more, less, or an equal share of the earth's resources. Our actions lead to amiable relations or to combative ones.

Here are some ideas for helping develop social judgment.

- Truly understand that whole grains are an appropriate principal food for humanity.
- Accept and respect the uniqueness of each person.
- Develop a sense of purpose in life that includes the mutual welfare of all living beings.
- Affirm, embody, express, unveil, and disseminate empowerment to yourself and others.
- Welcome empathy.

These activities can lead us to greater fellowship with others. We can become more considerate. As we welcome our cooperative responsibility for living in accord with others, we increase our social judgment, leading to Unconditional Love.

Sixth Judgment: Ideological

Ideological judgment is characterized by theoretical, conceptual, or religious thinking and justice. It includes the ability to distinguish and understand good from bad and right from wrong from a philosophical perspective. Ideological judgment usually begins around the age of twenty.

This judgment leads to a set of principles that are formed and adopted by each of us. We use these principles to judge the merits of the decisions we make. Often we include the doctrines of various philosophers, theologians, friends, and family members along with one or several philosophical or religious organizations. These theoretical concepts are shaped by our own innate sense of what is right and what is wrong.

We live in a world of polarization or sides. It is easy to accept one side while denying the other. Such an approach leads us toward dualistic thinking and away from wholeness. In order to unify those things that appear to us as opposites, we need to accept or embrace both sides as one. Here are some ideas for consideration:

- Learn how to change the quality of foods through dialectical or macrobiotic cooking.
- Realize that everything is constantly changing during our lifetimes.
- Embrace both sides of all apparent opposites.
- Understand that even though each of us is unique in appearance, we are connected or one in spirit.
- Develop true faith that allows union with the Infinite.

These activities can help us develop a sense of wholeness and meaning in our lives. We can become more fair in our dealings with others. We can develop the capacity to realign our thinking whenever needed. In these ways we can accept and embody absolute justice.

Seventh Judgment: Supreme

Supreme Judgment is unveiled when we embrace all opposites and realize universal unification with the Infinite. In fact, Supreme Judgment is another name for the Infinite or Oneness. The six other judgments begin at sometime. The seventh judgment is with us always—it is all-powerful and unsurpassed. This judgment becomes unveiled to us as we strengthen, develop, and increase the six other judgments.

Ohsawa compares these judgments to the growth of a tree. Physical judgment is like the roots, adapting themselves as required pretty much out of sight and mind. Sensory judgment is like the bark, carrying nourishment in all directions. Sentimental judgment is like the trunk, providing support or stability for the entire tree. Intellectual judgment is like the branches, filling out the tree in a balanced or correct way. Social judgment is like the leaves, each expressing its uniqueness while collecting the sun's nourishment. Intellectual judgment is like the flowers and fruit, showing and providing the tree's meaning or reason to be.

In this analogy, Supreme Judgment is like the seed that contains the blueprint for the entire tree, the entire tree itself, and the Infinite space contained within the tree. Mr. Masanobu Fukuoka, author of *One-Straw Revolution* and *The Natural Way of Farming* explained the difference between the finite and the Infinite. He drew a big circle on the chalkboard that he identified as a bubble. He explained that we are in the bubble as long as we see anything as separate from anything else. Learning to see opposites and to unify them is helpful, yet we remain in the bubble. In order to experience the Infinite or Oneness, we must get to the point that we don't see any opposites or any separation whatsoever. In other words, as long as we see the bubble we are in the bubble.

The Infinite is not only surrounding the bubble, but also is within the bubble. There is only one Infinite, and thus everything is part of the Infinite. Within the bubble, we are bound by time and space. The

Infinite is not limited by time and space. We experience the Infinite within the bubble as moments of Grace, inspiration, or intuition.

Moments of Grace, inspiration, or intuition come to us regardless of what we do. We do not need to eat certain foods and avoid others. Study of macrobiotic principles is not required. Religious or spiritual practices are unnecessary. Each person has the same capacity within. However, strengthening, developing, and increasing each of the judgments through macrobiotic practice is beneficial.

During moments of Grace, inspiration, or intuition, the more adaptive our physical judgment, the more open we can be to them. The more sensitive our sensorial judgment, the more such moments nurture us. The more stable our sentimental judgment, the more expressive we can be with our feelings. The more insightful and honest our intellectual judgment, the more awareness we can allow ourselves. The greater our social judgment, the more loving we can be. The greater our ideological judgment, the greater the meaning such moments have.

Because we are human, we must not forget the backside however. The more we receive, the more our egos grow. We begin to think we are responsible—that the ideas are ours. We become arrogant. This can lead to sickness. Often, it is during times of great sickness that great insights come. Supreme Judgment may be realized.

At this level of understanding or judgment, we can eat and drink anything with great pleasure and without fear. We embody complete happiness. We can realize our true Self, putting aside our limited egos. We can understand Life with crystal clarity. We can embrace every one and every thing. We can fulfill all our dreams throughout life. We can be totally free.

Conclusion

For purposes of analysis, Ohsawa separated judgment or consciousness into seven stages or levels. In reality, there is only one judgment with various aspects just as there is one tree with roots, bark, trunk, branches, leaves and flowers, fruit, and seeds. Strengthening, developing, and increasing all aspects of our judgment can lead to greater health, happiness, peace, wisdom, love, justice, and freedom in our lives. We can transform any difficult time in a positive way. We can turn pain and suffering from the death of a loved one to understanding and joy through an understanding of the stages of judgment.

In addition to our mourning and sorrow, we can increase our physical adaptability and become more creative and open. In addition to our sadness and tears, we can increase the sensitivity of our senses and become more nurturing and giving. In addition to our pain and anguish, we can increase our emotional stability and become more grateful and realize more of our potential. In addition to our analyzing and complaining, we can increase our intellectual clarity and become more honest and allow greater awareness. In addition to our faultfinding and heartaches, we can increase our social empathy and become more expressive and accepting. In addition to our distress and regret, we can increase our ideological meaning and become more unifying and have greater faith. In addition to our despair and suffering over loss, we can increase our supreme inspiration and become more intuitive, and can realize Oneness within ourselves and with others.

Macrobiotic Healing

In macrobiotic thinking, health is a condition of living in dynamic balance between yin and yang. In health, the movements between yin and yang are easy and smooth. Sickness is a condition of imbalance occurring when the changes between yin and yang are more difficult and rough, or when there is a blockage of movement between them. Healing is the process of going from an unbalanced condition to a more balanced one. It is most important to understand that there is no perfect balance—yin or yang is always in excess in every thing, in every person, and at every time. Thus, healing is an ongoing process and everyone is constantly healing. In times of health, the interplay between yin and yang is hardly noticed but it is there just the same. In times of sickness, one recognizes the need for change more readily.

Macrobiotic principles are used in an attempt to stay in the balanced area of health as much of the time as possible and to minimize both the time and severity of any imbalance. Changes in the season, climate, diet, environment, stress levels, and all of life requires adjustments in order to accomplish this goal. The macrobiotic way is to allow the body's own healing power to work by avoiding overburdening the system with excesses or extreme foods. This is done by using a macrobiotic centering diet, by using the principles of yin and yang, or by using any of a number of natural home remedies. These methods are explained in detail in this chapter.

Macrobiotic healing is not medicine; it uses no medication or surgery. Macrobiotic healing methods may be used along with other therapies, including medical intervention, but this is beyond the scope of this book. Other holistic approaches such as homeopathy, naturopathy, Ayurvedic, and traditional Chinese medicine that take into account the whole person rather than just the disease symptoms work well with the macrobiotic approach. If a person chooses such a course of action, seeking the advice of a qualified macrobiotic counselor or care provider is recommended.

No matter how one lives and deals with life's changes, the body will wear out eventually. Macrobiotic practice strives to make the most of each person's constitution, giving them a longer and healthier life than they might enjoy otherwise. While death is inevitable, the manner in which one dies varies greatly. The possibility of dying in one's sleep of natural causes (the body simply wearing out) and not of a major disease is one of the objectives of macrobiotic living.

Looking more closely at health and sickness, just as there is a natural order to life and health, there is a natural order or progression to sickness. In order to maintain a healthy physical condition, most internal body conditions must remain fairly constant. Examples include the pH level of the blood, blood sugar levels, internal body temperature, oxygen and carbon dioxide levels, and so on. As long as balanced internal conditions are maintained, health is the result. When balanced internal conditions are not maintained, sickness is the result.

Sickness is the body's warning that there is an imbalance, and thus can be viewed as the body's natural attempt to maintain balanced internal conditions. If the warning is heeded and taken care of in a natural way, health returns quickly. If the warning is unheeded or taken care of in an unnatural way, the body must take more extreme measures to maintain balanced internal conditions. The sickness gets progressively more severe and the remedy takes longer and can be more difficult.

This chapter contains an explanation of the stages of sickness from a macrobiotic viewpoint as developed by George Ohsawa and Herman Aihara. Within the stages, while there are usually immediate causes of any new difficulty, the underlying root cause is the same—an excess of yin or yang or both. Stage one and stage two sicknesses are transitory in nature, while stages three through five are chronic conditions that require greater care. The sooner any imbalance is remedied the better.

The chapter continues with a section on macrobiotic centering diets and diagnosis, showing that often a simple natural diet is the best approach to healing. The section on the process of macrobiotic healing explains what to expect if dietary changes are made. Natural home remedies that are supplemental and may be used for relief of symptoms are explained next. The chapter concludes with a section on some of the factors in health other than food, although examples both of non-food causes and non-food remedies can be found throughout this chapter on the stages of sickness.

Stages of Sickness

Stage 1: Fatigue. As with many disorders and sicknesses these days, fatigue is seen as a natural occurrence rather than as a sickness. However, from a macrobiotic perspective, fatigue is the first sign of sickness. If the fatigue is understood and dealt with in a natural way, more serious sickness can be avoided. There are many causes of fatigue and dulled mental awareness, including:

- Too much acidity in the body.
- Any reduction in the oxygen supply to the cells, such as too much fat in the blood, a low red blood cell count, or low blood sugar.
- Poor circulation from a lack of exercise. Too much strenuous exercise also causes fatigue.
- Elimination disorders, such as constipation or diarrhea.
- Overworking, overeating, or too much stress.

Any fatigue is a sign that the body, and especially the organs, are having to work too much. Sometimes a brief rest or a vacation is all that is needed. In other cases, more must be done. Here are some ways to counteract fatigue or dulled mental awareness.

- Breathe deeply and completely, concentrating on the exhalation. This helps increase the amount of oxygen and decrease the amount of carbon dioxide in the body. Put your hands on the front and back of your abdomen just below your belt. This area should move outward in both the front and the back when you breathe in. Learn to breathe so this area moves outward when inhaling.

- Chew your food well. Eat less if fatigue comes from overeating and your body can handle eating less.
- Improve blood circulation by taking hot foot baths, alternating hot and cold showers if your body can handle the shock, or by exercising. Do exercises that elevate the heart rate as your condition allows.
- Avoid strenuous exercise if that is the cause of your fatigue or if your condition does not allow it. Walking, gardening, Do-In self massage, and other mild circulation-enhancing exercises are helpful.
- Apply ginger compresses over the kidneys.
- Consume more alkaline-forming and less acid-forming foods and drinks. This is better than taking antacid pills.
- Take cool showers or baths. Hot baths are more acid-forming.
- Learn to control tension in your body. Any kind of meditation or muscle relaxing technique is helpful.
- Become more open and honest with your feelings. This helps by reducing stress.
- Live within your limits. Every child knows when to stop, but adults often do too much. Learn what you can and can't effectively influence and act accordingly.

Stage 2: Aches and pain. If fatigue or dulled mental awareness is not dealt with in a natural way, the next stage is pain, often in the form of headaches. Also, a state of fatigue makes one more vulnerable to injuries that result in various kinds of pain.

Pain is a warning that something is wrong and needs attention. In cases of injury such as a cut or a bruise, one deals with the pain and tries not to let the same thing happen again. However, most people suffer from little aches and pains that they have learned to live with. These are also warnings that something is wrong. The modern response is to stop the pain. The macrobiotic response is to determine the cause of the pain and then to deal with that cause. Both responses get rid of the pain; however, the modern response does nothing to remedy the cause of the pain, and the sickness progresses to the next stage.

Almost every injury or sickness has pain associated with it. According to Herman Aihara, the actual cause of the pain is a shortage of oxygen in the nerve cells. For example, a shortage of oxygen in the brain leads to a headache. Taking aspirin or other headache medication stops the pain by shutting down the warning system. It's similar to killing the messenger who brings bad news. Taking drugs is more dangerous than the pain—most painkillers also damage the nervous system and often lead to more severe illness. It is far better to learn how to deal with the pain in a more natural way.

The most lasting relief from recurring aches and pains—from headaches to stiff shoulders to back pain to foot pains—is a change to a macrobiotic approach to diet and lifestyle. Achieving such relief can take weeks to years, depending on the depth of the underlying sickness. Here are some common natural remedies for temporary relief of pain.

- A ginger compress applied to the affected area increases the circulation of blood to that area and gives temporary relief from pain. An albi plaster is often used immediately after a ginger compress.
- A tofu plaster is usually used on the head, and green plasters are useful for milder pains on either the head or the body.
- Massaging the painful area is helpful, especially for headaches.
- Various teas, including sho-ban tea and umesho bancha tea, are useful.

See the chapter on natural home remedies for instructions on making and applying many of the remedies listed here. Consult *Natural Healing from Head to Toe* by Cornellia and Herman Aihara or a similar book for additional useful home remedies.

Stage 3: Infections and infectious diseases. The next stage of sickness is infections and infectious diseases. Many microbes live within the body. These microbes aid in digestion and metabolism, and are necessary for a healthy life. When the natural order is not followed, unhealthy microbes can grow and cause inflammation, swelling, itching, and pain, damaging healthy cells. The most dangerous microbes can survive without oxygen and therefore are harder for the body's immune system to deal with. Problems occur most frequently when there are too many microbes in the body. The environment that causes microbes to grow excessively is produced by any or all of the following conditions.

- Too much simple sugar, such as from refined sugar or fruit.
- Excess water or liquid intake.
- Excessive amounts of protein.
- Too little sodium.
- A warm environment or season. (Unhealthy microbes have trouble living in too cold or too hot an environment).

These conditions all lead to an overly yin condition and a weakened immune system. Winter is the most yin season. An overly yin diet in the winter leads to a greater chance to develop a cold. The natural remedy for these conditions that encourage the growth of microbes is quite simple. Avoid simple sugars, excessive liquid or protein intake, and use enough sea salt in cooking to ensure an adequate amount of sodium in the body fluids. A macrobiotic diet meets all these requirements perfectly. In addition to the home remedies discussed in this book, the topical applications as discussed in Natural Healing from Head to Toe can bring natural relief from inflammation, swelling, itching, or other symptoms associated with infections.

The modern typical approach is to stop the symptoms; for example, taking aspirin for a fever. According to macrobiotic thinking, a fever is not only the body's warning that something is wrong, but also the body's natural attempt to deal with excessive unhealthy microbes or bacteria by creating an environment that is too hot for them. Stopping the fever only allows the microbes to get an even stronger hold, leading to deeper diseases. The macrobiotic approach is to let the fever run its course unless the temperature rises too high (over 103 degrees). In this case, natural remedies are used to reduce the fever to a manageable temperature and then to let it finish running its course.

Another modern typical approach to infections is antibiotics. Here again the response is to kill the messenger rather than dealing with the underlying cause. Antibiotics do stop the symptoms of infections and are often referred to as wonder drugs. The overall effect on the immune system is not positive however. With antibiotics many infectious diseases have been "cured" miraculously. As stronger and stronger infectious diseases have developed because the bacteria become resistant to the antibiotics, newer and stronger antibiotic drugs have followed. The reason for the stronger diseases in the first place is that the use of antibiotics weakens the body's immune system, contributing to the development of diseases such as candida, environmental sensitivities or illnesses, herpes, AIDS, and many more. Here again the response is to kill the messenger rather than dealing with the underlying cause.

Stage 4: Autonomic nervous system. Ignoring or destroying the body's warning signals and eating poorly eventually weaken the autonomic nervous system. The result is problems with hormone secretions and the proper functioning of the organs. This is another result of an overly acidic diet, which slows first nerve cell function and then hormone secretions. Problems with insulin, cortical hormone, and thyroid gland secretions are examples of the results of a long-term diet of too much fatty animal foods, sugary foods, processed foods, and foods containing chemicals.

Diabetes, one of the leading causes of death in the United States, is a good example of the fourth stage of sickness. There are two types of diabetes, insulin-dependent and non-insulin-dependent, but in both cases the problem is insufficient insulin. Frequent urination, constant thirst, weight loss despite eating a lot of food, cramps, blurred vision, and feeling tired and run-down all the time are some of the symptoms of insulin-dependent diabetes. According to macrobiotic thinking, the underlying cause is a diet that includes too much sweet food and drinks, including fruits and fruit juices. These foods cause the beta cells that produce insulin to be weakened so that not enough insulin is produced. Another underlying cause is too much fat in the diet. In this case, the body may be able to make insulin but neither insulin nor glucose can pass through the membranes of either blood vessels or cells because of the excess fat. The cells die from starvation. Non-insulin-dependent diabetes is similar, except that overconsumption of fatty foods is the major underlying cause.

The natural home remedies chapter and books such as *Natural Healing from Head to Toe* provide remedies for the symptoms associated with diabetes and other nervous system disorders, but only a change to a more natural way of eating such as a macrobiotic diet or macrobiotic centering diet allows the body to return to its natural healthy condition. Injections or stimulants and depressants used to control hormonal secretions are not the answer. They do nothing to remedy the underlying cause, and only serve to drive the sickness deeper into the cells and organs.

Stage 5a: Organ diseases. These are the life-threatening diseases such as heart disease and cancer. Here is a brief introduction to macrobiotic thinking regarding heart disease, as an example of organ diseases.

Even though the percentage of deaths from heart disease has decreased due to a greater understanding of the role of fats and cholesterol, heart disease is still the leading cause of death in the United States. Fats and cholesterol narrow the artery walls, restricting blood flow and limiting the amount of oxygen available to the heart. In the case of a heart attack, the lack of oxygen causes pain, and if action is not taken quickly enough, death is often the result. The modern response is to use drugs to control the amount of cholesterol and triglycerides, another type of blood fat. If this doesn't work, surgery to clear the blockage is often the next or only option.

According to macrobiotic thinking, the underlying causes and risk factors that contribute to heart attacks are:

- A diet high in fat and cholesterol from animal food sources.
- A diet high in simple sugars, including fruit sugar. Excess simple sugars easily turn to fat in the body.
- Too much or too little salt. Too little salt weakens the body's ability to make white blood cells and thus weakens the immune system. Too much salt can lead to kidney problems, and too much salt in conjunction with too much fat leads to high blood pressure.
- Smoking, stress, or obesity.
- Overwork, fatigue, or a sedentary lifestyle.

The macrobiotic approach is to deal with the underlying causes of heart disease. A macrobiotic diet—a balanced diet that is low in fat and protein from animal food sources and in simple sugars, and high in complex carbohydrates—is a good preventative for heart disease. Of course, people who have had a heart attack or who have any advanced heart disorder must deal with it quickly—a change in diet and lifestyle simply may take too much time. After medical intervention, however, a change in diet and lifestyle is definitely the best option.

Stage 5b: Cell diseases. Organs and cells work together closely. Organs, of course, are made up of cells. And one of the main functions of the organs is to maintain constant conditions for the body fluids, such as the blood and cellular fluids, that make cells healthy. If the body fluid is not healthy, the cells become sick and the organs become weaker. Weak organs cannot maintain constant conditions for the body fluids, so the cells become weaker, and so on. Here is a brief introduction to macrobiotic thinking regarding cancer, the worst-case example of cell sickness.

According to Herman Aihara, cancer (the malignant growth of cells) begins as a result of overly acidic body fluids. The blood needs to be slightly alkaline, with a pH from 7.35 to 7.45. The organs, and especially the kidneys, filter out acids to maintain such an alkaline condition. The over-consumption of acid-forming foods and fats leads to overworked and weakened kidneys.

The underlying cause of cancer is a diet or lifestyle that produces too much acid. A diet of animal foods (especially fatty meats), simple sugars and sugary foods, and synthetic chemicals such as flavorings, colorings, preservatives, and conditioners can cause cancer. The metabolism of fat creates large amounts of acid wastes, and fats slow blood circulation. The metabolism of simple sugar increases the level of carbon dioxide, leading to an acidic condition. Simple sugars also destroy red blood cells. Fruits are alkaline-forming; however, they are more yin and further weaken an already weakened immune system. And because fruit sugar readily changes to fat in the body, avoiding fruits is usually recommended by macrobiotic counselors for those with cancer.

Animal protein, animal fat, and simple sugars also help the cancer cells grow and thrive. The macrobiotic approach to cancer is to avoid these foods and follow a diet low in fat and simple sugars. Cancer cells cannot grow without excessive amounts of these nutrients; they eventually die without developing new cancer cells. Many other substances, such as known carcinogens, x-rays, atomic radiation, and asbestos, also contribute to the development of cancer. As in the case of heart disease, people who have an advanced cancer (for example, the cancer cells are strong and growing quickly) should consider medical or alternative intervention because the macrobiotic approach may take too much time.

The role of the kidneys is so very important in all fifth-stage disorders, and most people have weakened kidneys from the advice to drink as much as one can. Here are some ways to strengthen the kidneys—any one or all are helpful. See the chapter on natural home remedies for instructions.

- Follow a macrobiotic dietary approach, which does not require large amounts of excess liquid.
- Apply a ginger compress over the kidney area for twenty minutes each day for at least one month. Continue as needed.
- Walk barefoot on the grass in the early morning for five to ten minutes every day.
- Take two or three salt baths per week in a 1 percent salt solution (one pound of any kind of salt in twelve gallons of water) for about twenty minutes per bath.

Stage 6: Psychological sicknesses. Psychological sicknesses or imbalances are another warning signal that changes in diet and lifestyle need to be made. While physical sicknesses generally follow a pattern from stage 1 to stage 5, psychological imbalances can happen at any time and can trigger or greatly contribute to physical sickness. Conversely, a physical sickness can trigger or greatly contribute to psychological sickness. Psychological imbalances themselves follow a natural progression or order. For example, feelings can be positive or negative. Positive feelings are alkaline-forming, add to one's sense of strength, and lead to more energy. Negative feelings are acid-forming, use up energy, and lead to fatigue.

During each person's life there are times of loss, from the loss of friendships, to the loss of a job, to the death of a spouse or relative. Anxiety is the fear of hurt or loss. Hurt, loss, or anxiety over loss all lead to pain. If one grieves for the original loss near the time of the loss, a return to psychological balance is the result. Any pain left inside demands a response of energy that is directed outward and is usually expressed as anger. Anger held in leads to guilt, and unrelieved guilt leads to depression, a disruption of the flow of feelings that consumes all energy. In other words, the imbalance of emotions progresses until it is dealt with in a natural open and honest way or until it becomes so severe that it completely overwhelms you. Physical sickness or food imbalances make it more difficult to deal with any psychological imbalance. Physical sickness itself is a loss—the loss of health. Thus, physical sicknesses and psychological imbalances often feed on each other. Here are some warning signals that show psychological imbalance.

- Not wanting to get up in the morning or feeling that little can be done to change one's life. A healthy person is full of motivation to get up and work each day and knows all problems can be solved sooner or later.
- Blaming oneself for a long time for failures or disappointments. Everyone fails at times. A healthy person can deal with failures or disappointments quickly and honestly.
- Feeling that plans will turn out badly, that planned events will be canceled, or shying away from difficult tasks out of fear of failure. A healthy person is positive about the future and does not shy away from difficult tasks.
- Always looking to others for cures of even minor symptoms. A healthy person lets the body's own healing power remedy such symptoms. Always taking medications or always going to the doctor is a sign of imbalance. Doing whatever someone else says out of a fear of taking responsibility for one's decisions is a sign of deeper imbalance.
- Paranoia. A healthy person is instinctively afraid of crazy or threatening people, but a fear of everyone is a signal of imbalance.
- Often feeling alienated or separated from others, or having few close relationships. A healthy person fits in with others and has close friends with whom to share failures or temporary unhappiness.
- Difficulty showing anger. A healthy person is able to express anger appropriately in a non-threatening way when necessary.

Most of these conditions are a result of a diet that is too yin. For example, it may include too many simple sugars. A change in diet can be most helpful in restoring balance to one's emotional and psychological condition. Creating the space, time, privacy, and peace to get in touch with and to be open and honest about one's feelings daily is very helpful as well.

Stage 7: Spiritual sickness. A spiritually healthy person has faith in oneness, the natural order of life; takes responsibility for all his or her actions; is not exclusive; lives with infinite gratitude and appreciation for life. A lack of faith and a lack of appreciation for the oneness of life is spiritual sickness—the deepest sickness of all. This is the beginning of the dualistic thinking that sees enemies and leads to an unhappy life of fear. For example, modern medicine sees unhealthy microbes and cancer cells as enemies that must be killed before they kill us. The macrobiotic understanding is that all so-called "enemies" exist to help us understand the natural order of life. Thus, unhealthy microbes and cancer cells are part of us, and therefore are part of the world of oneness. They are necessary warning signals. A person who understands that unhealthy microbes and cancer cells are a blessing because they help show the cause of such a condition is well on the way to a natural healthy life.

Ohsawa outlined seven judging abilities to show people how to regain spiritual health as described in the section on Macrobiotic Theory, pages 65-74. A person who reaches the seventh ability, supreme judgment, can unify all opposites. Hate changes to love, enemy changes to friend, sickness changes to health, unhappiness changes to happiness. Such a person has absolute faith, has no fear, and can maintain peace of mind, leading to eternal happiness. A person who truly understands and possesses supreme judgment can cure any sickness easily and naturally by allowing the body's healing power to remedy any disorder.

Macrobiotic Centering Diet and Diagnosis

Most diseases in civilized society come from excesses rather than from deficiencies. The macrobiotic way of expressing this is too much yin, too much yang, too much extreme yin and yang, or too much acid-forming food. (Cases involving too much alkaline-forming food are very rare.) In simple cases a dietary remedy is easy: simply eat more foods with the opposite qualities and fewer foods with the same quality.

However, many cases are more complex. Nothing in this world, including one's condition, is ever all yin or all yang. Just as with categorizing foods, all the yin characteristics and yang characteristics of a condition must be added up to determine if someone is overly yin or overly yang. There may be swelling (more yin) and redness (more yang) and so on. Adding up all the factors and deciding how much weight to give each one can be confusing.

Fortunately, simply eating a basic macrobiotic diet helps to restore the body's own healing power. One approach to healing is to eat a variety of foods when healthy and to use a beginning macrobiotic centering diet when sick or uncomfortable for any reason. This approach is used for short periods of time and is often all that is needed to restore health depending on the sickness (overly yin conditions respond best) and the strength of a person's natural healing power.

A macrobiotic centering diet is a restricted basic macrobiotic diet, eating and drinking only what is necessary for one's life, and toward the center of yin and yang balance. This means eating primarily whole grains, vegetables, beans, and sea vegetables. Sea salt either by itself or in miso, soy sauce, umeboshi, or gomashio, and liquid, usually bancha tea (kukicha), are also needed. Everything else is kept to a minimum or avoided altogether. This approach allows the body's natural healing power to heal from within.

For a macrobiotic centering diet, the percentage of whole grains is increased to 60 to 80 percent daily and pressure-cooked brown rice is usually the largest portion of this amount, although a variety of other whole grains may be used. If digestion of whole grains is a problem, or if a pressure cooker is not used, brown rice cream is recommended. This is whole brown rice roasted in a dry pan, ground, and then made into a porridge. Any of the less yang and less yin vegetables listed in the beginning macrobiotic diet chapter are eaten daily, totaling from 20 to 30 percent by volume. The extremely yin vegetables are avoided and of the more yin vegetables, leafy greens and broccoli are eaten most often.

Beans, primarily miso, natural soy sauce, aduki beans, chick-peas, and lentils, comprise from 3 to 10 percent daily. Of the sea vegetables, wakame, kombu, and hijiki are used most, from 3 to 5 percent of daily intake. One to two bowls of soup, usually miso soup, using the vegetables, grains, beans, and sea vegetables listed above are included in a centering diet. Bancha twig tea is used as one's primary beverage. Other teas found in the natural home remedy chapter are used for specific purposes.

Of the condiments, gomashio (ground roasted sesame seeds and sea salt) is used most. It, and any of the more yang condiments, are used as desired. Any of the more yang or less yin seasonings are used in small amounts for flavoring or to balance dishes. Of the oils, sesame oil is preferred, used sparingly. All of the supplemental foods, fruit, nuts, seeds, fish, and sweeteners, are avoided until one is better.

Quality becomes even more important with a macrobiotic centering diet. One should obtain the best water and the most organi-cally-grown foods possible. Chewing each mouthful of food at least one-hundred times is recommended so that the body spends less en-ergy breaking down food and more energy on the healing process. Overeating is avoided for the same reason.

This diet is to macrobiotic healing what a basic macrobiotic diet is to a macrobiotic dietary approach. It is a beginning simplified diet that can be used for general healing for ten days to two weeks or lon-ger, as long as one is benefiting from it. A complete remedy may take longer, requiring the next step—the introduction of yin and yang principles. Once a person is well it is important to widen the diet to include a greater variety of foods.

Developing a working knowledge of yin and yang, which pro-vides a greater understanding of the natural order of life, gives one greater control over the healing process. To begin, one adjusts the basic macrobiotic dietary approach, or the macrobiotic centering diet, based on the yin and yang qualities of foods eaten in the past and on one's present yin or yang condition of the body, emphasizing either yin or yang foods, as appropriate. Many of the guidelines needed for these adjustments are included in the section on macrobiotic yin and yang. If one makes a mistake and uses yin when yang is needed, the body keeps issuing warning signals, and the remedy can be changed. Nonetheless, to remedy a specific ailment using yin and yang, it may be necessary to consult a book or someone with more experience. Either increases one's understanding of yin and yang.

The rest of this chapter presents some of the conditions that signal that a change of diet is needed. Most of these warning signals rely on the principle that the condition outside reflects the condition inside. In addition, the chapter briefly mentions some of the disciplines studied by practitioners of macrobiotic diagnosis—a field that is far too detailed and complex to cover fully here.

Here are some useful diagnosis tools for each organ. They show an imbalance and an actual or impending sickness if corrective measures are not taken.

Lungs: An overall white or pale skin color indicates lung trouble, as does excessive yawning. Frequent headaches, melancholy, or depression may indicate insufficient oxygen in the brain due to poor lung functioning.

Large intestine: Evacuating more or less frequently than once a day (or a person's normal amount) or bad odor in the feces may signal a problem with the large intestines. If the feces are shrunken and dry, it indicates too much salt. If the feces have no shape, it indicates too little salt plus an excess of milk, fruit, or simple sugars. An easy test is to walk barefoot on stones—pain indicates poor functioning of the digestive organs, including the large intestine and the kidneys.

Stomach: A blue line along the inside or at the base of the thumb, a white tongue, and chapped lips (except as a normal changing of the skin) are signals of possible stomach problems. A thick upper lip indicates overeating, especially sugary yin foods and refined foods.

A cyst on the lips shows over-acidity in the stomach and a possible ulcer.

Spleen/pancreas: Malfunctioning of the spleen/pancreas is shown by yellowish skin, cracked feet, excessive sleeping during the day, anemia, dull legs, or cravings for sweets. Forgetfulness and over-worry indicate spleen trouble, which is usually the result of eating too much sweet foods.

Heart: The tip of the nose shows the condition of the heart. A purple color or puffiness indicates a weak over-expanded heart, usually from too much alcoholic drink or fruit juice. A red color shows an inflamed heart and possible high blood pressure. An oily or shiny condition shows an excess of animal protein. A red tongue or a large deep crack down the middle of the tongue is another indicator of possible heart problems.

Small intestine: An expanded lower lip indicates the overeating of fatty foods and problems with the intestines. Pimples and rashes indicate an excess of toxins in the body, usually from the overcon-sumption of animal foods. Stiff shoulders or trouble turning the head from side to side indicates possible small intestine problems.

Urinary bladder: Frequent urination that is dark or black indicates a contracted bladder. Other bladder problem indicators are sensitiv-ity to cold and wind, itchy running eyes, and pain in the neck, back-bone, kidney area, or ankles. If the vessels on the back of the hands are bulging or if there is pain when the back of one hand is slapped by the fingers of the other hand, the body has too much liquid. Wa-tery eyes, a runny nose, or sneezing also signal too much liquid.

Kidneys: Bags or puffiness under the eyes indicate weak kidneys. Dark brown or black color under the eyes indicates overly yang kid-neys, as does dark urine or a shrunken small toe with a very small nail. Athlete's foot comes from bad kidneys, as a result of too much animal protein. Other indicators of weak (overly yin) kidneys are light-colored urine or frequent urination that is like water, along with cold feet. The ears and skin also show the condition of the kidneys; any ear or skin problem indicates that the kidneys need help. In all cases, control liquid and salt intake and avoid animal foods.

Circulation/sex (heart governor): Dark lips or coldness in the hands or feet show poor blood circulation, usually from excess animal foods and strong yin foods such as simple sugar. A horizontal line between the mouth and the nose indicates a malfunction of the sexual organs. Swelling in the armpits, constant thirst, and rancid-smelling breath are further indicators of heart governor problems.

Pituitary/hormonal system (triple warmer): Trembling hands or fingers indicates a problem with the triple warmer, as does significantly different temperatures between the top and bottom parts of the body (such as constantly being cold from the waist up while warm from the waist down).

Gallbladder: Swelling around the upper eyelids shows the possibility of gallstones. Yellow palms on the hands indicates a problem with the gallbladder along with the spleen/pancreas and possibly the liver.

Liver: Lines between the eyebrows indicate liver problems and that a person is temperamental. Vertical lines show that the overworked liver is in a more yin condition, and reveal a tendency toward complaining. A horizontal line between the eyebrows shows a more yang liver, and reveals a tendency toward anger. A red color in the whites of the eyes indicates the overconsumption of food, especially fatty animal foods. Visible blue blood capillaries, dry throat, or the inability to bend forward or backward also indicate possible liver trouble.

Many of these indicators of organ trouble may be visible at the beginning of a person's macrobiotic practice. Others may develop as the body removes toxins and returns to health. The interrelationship between the organs and certain parts of the body comes from the theory of five elements, an ancient Chinese system reported to be over four thousand years old. In this system each of five fundamental elements are given a direction, season, yang organ, yin organ, emotion, grain, vegetable, and a host of other classifications. With study one can determine the best foods to strengthen each organ.

Just as there is a system of arteries and veins carrying blood throughout the body, there is also a system of meridians that carries energy through the body. This is the system used by acupuncturists to control and change one's condition using needles. The same system is used in Do-In self-massage for similar purposes. The meridians follow definite paths through the body and all pass through one of the fingers or one of the toes. Moving and massaging each finger and each toe every morning stimulates all of the organs. Moving all the joints from the fingers to the toes and tapping the bottom of each foot with the opposite fist every day is also beneficial to all the organs.

Here are some ideas on the yin and yang of organs. Again, the macrobiotic usage is different from traditional Chinese (Oriental) Medicine. The organs are paired in terms of function so that one organ is more yin, and one is more yang. There are two "organs" that are used in traditional Chinese Medicine, acupuncture, and Do-In that are not used in Western medicine. One is called the "heart governor" and is often referred to as "circulation/sex." The other is the "triple warmer" and is often referred to as "pituitary/hormonal system." Here are the yin and yang organ pairs and the corresponding fingers and toes where their meridians either begin or end.

Yin and Yang of Organs

more yang	more yin
kidneys (little toe/ bottom of foot)	urinary bladder (little toe)
liver (big toe)	gallbladder (fourth toe)
heart (little finger)	small intestines (little finger)

spleen/pancreas (big toe)	stomach (second and third toes)
lungs (thumb)	large intestines (index finger)
heart governor (second finger)	triple warmer (third finger)

While all the organs are important for a healthy body, the more yang organs are necessary for any life at all. In other words, a person can survive for longer without the more yin organs. The more yin organs work and then they rest, whereas the more yang organs are always working. It is important to let the yin organs rest. One of their functions is to protect the yang organs; a problem with a yang organ indicates a prior problem with the corresponding yin organ. For example, a person with a lung problem should look for ways to strengthen the large intestine as well as the lungs.

In using the meridian system, one learns that all the organ energies are connected. Sickness may be viewed as an imbalance in this energy system resulting from an excess or deficiency in one or more organs, often a blockage of the energy flow. Knowing where the meridians are can be useful in diagnosis of a condition. For example, a second toe that is longer than the big toe shows an overly expanded stomach, and thus a tendency toward a weak stomach. Redness or pain in a finger or toe would indicate a problem with the corresponding organ. Again, the basic principle is that the outside condition reflects the condition inside. Similarly, the face, eyes, ears, teeth, and feet are examples of more visible parts that reflect the condition of the inside.

The Process of Macrobiotic Healing

Just as there is a natural order to life and health and a natural order to or progression in sickness, there is also a natural order for turning an unhealthy body to a healthy one. This chapter explains how people who are using or changing to a macrobiotic approach move from sickness to health. Of course, every individual is different and will experience different results.

Healing always occurs in three stages. Any change to a more natural diet and lifestyle begins with a temporary worsening of the body's condition as it discharges toxins. This occurs as the body's natural healing power gets stronger from not having to deal with excesses or additional toxin-producing substances. The usual order is from yang to yin, or more specifically in the following order: meat, cheese, excessive fruit, dairy, alcohol, refined sugar, and drugs. It's clear what is being discharged because cravings, sometimes intense cravings, accompany the elimination. The discharge process may last for days, weeks, or longer. Discharges vary greatly from intense, dramatic events to slower, more tame affairs depending on the substances being discharged, the severity of the imbalance, and the length of time the body has been unbalanced. Still, one should expect some level of temporary discomfort. It almost always involves some pain, usually beginning in the neck and traveling downward through the body to the fingertips and toes and upward to the top of the head. Pain will be felt also in any weak or malfunctioning organs. A person undergoing a discharge may appear quite sick, but is often happy, especially if they understand the healing power.

The toxins may be expelled in any way possible, from the normal elimination channels of breathing, sweating, urinating, and defecating, to vomiting and discharges from the nose, ears, eyes, and reproductive organs. Green liquid bile and a colorless sticky substance from the intestines may come out. Black feces containing tiny stones are not uncommon. Massaging the naval area can help move old stagnant feces.

During the discharge process, white or yellow moles may appear at the back of the tongue that move toward the tip until they disappear, signaling a return to health. Black moles indicate the possibility of cancer. Redness on the body shows that the bloodstream is being cleansed. When the redness is only in the fingers and toes the discharge is about over. A headache often signals the end of a discharge and some people report seeing ghosts or visions at this time.

It is best to let the healing process finish naturally, but eating a small amount of the food being discharged will stop a discharge of toxins that is happening too rapidly and painfully. Medications and painkillers are not recommended; they can make the condition worse in the long run. Drinking less can hasten the discharge but will also increase the desire for foods and drinks that are being discharged. During a discharge, a simple diet of whole grains and fresh vegetables is best.

The second step in healing is to restore a healthy condition of the red blood cells. The red blood cells change completely every three months, becoming healthier very quickly. Most people who make a change to a macrobiotic dietary approach experience a marked improvement in health after the initial discharge period. Shortly after the change of red blood cells, the intercellular fluid (the fluid between cells) is changed. This time, usually the second to the fourth months, can be quite exhilarating. Many people feel that they have found the answer to healthy living.

The third step, however, is more gradual and can be much more difficult, and there may even be an occasional worsening of one's condition. This step is the healing of the rest of the body cells themselves. Nutritive substances from the improved intercellular fluid enter the cells and gradually make them healthier. However, most cells are not as adaptable to change as the red blood cells and the intercellular fluids. In other words, they do not easily adapt to the new intercellular fluid and while the benefits of new, more healthy body cells are on the horizon, another temporary weakening or worsening of condition is felt. This usually happens anywhere from the fourth month to several years after beginning a macrobiotic dietary approach. It is important to understand that this worsening of condition is a prelude to greater health.

Because the natural order is change, even after the first dramatic healing process has been completed, the body is continuously expelling toxins or excess materials or making adjustments and experiencing temporary worsenings of its condition. These are opportunities to increase one's understanding of the healing process. These are actually signs that one is in good health but must simply learn from experience and from solving new problems.

Natural Home Remedies

Simple home remedies made from foods can be helpful for people who have followed a macrobiotic approach to diet for a long time, as well as people just beginning a macrobiotic practice. Home remedies can bring relief from discomfort stemming from many causes, including: old toxins or undischarged excesses; toxic materials in houses, furniture, cosmetics, or polluted air; or too much stress.

The remedies in this chapter fit a macrobiotic approach because they are made of natural foods and contribute to the healing process. There are many other natural home remedies used within macrobiotic practice, and any natural food or drink, including medicinal herbs and herb teas from other holistic healing approaches, are used as needed or desired. However, the yin or yang effect of such remedies must be factored into the total healing process. In contrast, synthetic drugs, which tend to be extremely yin or extremely yang, frequently stop or hinder the healing process. However, no home remedy cures a disease; it can simply relieve symptoms and encourage healing.

Many of the preparations use ginger. This yin spice acts as a stimulant, boosting circulation and helping internal cleansing of the body. The remedies listed here also make use of ginger's ability to increase respiration, digestion, and nervous-system function. The Recommended Readings include a few books that discuss more home remedies.

—Ginger Sesame Oil—

Ginger sesame oil may be used for massaging any area, and is useful for headaches, dandruff, pain in the spine or joints, skin problems, or numbness. To help heal a curved spine, put the ginger sesame oil on the index and second fingers and massage down the spine with one finger on either side of the spine. Do this for about 30 minutes each time. This massage is very relaxing for anybody.

To make the ginger sesame oil, grate 1 to 2 teaspoons of fresh ginger with a fine Japanese grater (available from Asian markets, some natural food stores, or mail order suppliers). Squeeze the juice into a small bowl. Add an equal amount of sesame oil, and mix well. Any sesame oil will work, but pure dark sesame oil is best.

—Ginger Bath—

Freshly grated ginger juice added to your bath water is useful for improving blood circulation; relieving pain in the joints; itchiness, or other skin disorders; and for helping to remove old salts from the body. Ginger baths can be strong, and should be taken by adults only. Bring 20 cups of water to a boil and shut off the heat. For a medium-strength bath using fresh ginger, grate about ⅔ cup of ginger with a Japanese grater and put it in the middle of a square piece of cheesecloth. Bring the four corners together and tie them so that the ginger is inside. This is a "cheesecloth bag." Put the bag into the hot water. Do not boil the ginger, as this can reduce its effectiveness. After a few minutes, squeeze the bag with any utensil (such as a pair of chopsticks) so that all the ginger juice is expelled into the hot water. Place the ginger water in a bathtub and add enough warm water to cover the navel when lying down in the tub. Lie in this water for about 20 minutes. Use a greater proportion of ginger for a stronger bath or if the ginger is old. Decrease the proportion of ginger for a milder bath.

—Ginger Foot Bath—

This foot bath is good for improving blood circulation in general and for kidney disorders and insomnia in particular. Prepare the ginger water as for a ginger bath and put it in a pan. Soak the feet for about 10 minutes at a time.

—Ginger Compress—

The ginger compress is useful for any kind of pain, and when applied over the kidney area on the lower back is most helpful for strengthening the kidneys. It is simple, inexpensive, and very strong. Caution is suggested for severe disorders. Ginger compresses are not recommended for use on the breast in cases of breast cancer, on the head when there is high fever, or on the uterus area during pregnancy. It should not be used for appendicitis pain when there is fever, or on a baby. For an elderly person in a weakened condition, use a mild ginger compress (reduce the proportion of ginger juice) until the person's strength returns. Prepare ginger water as for a ginger bath, only using 10 cups of water and 1/3 cup of freshly grated ginger. The water may be reheated (do not bring to boil) and used again for up to 24 hours.

Dip a cotton or linen hand towel or other cotton cloth into the ginger water and squeeze out the excess water. (If your fingers are sensitive to the hot water, either wear rubber gloves or roll the towel lengthwise so you can put it in the ginger water without getting the ends wet.) Twist the towel by the ends, one end clockwise and the other counterclockwise, so that the excess water drips back into the pan. You need to keep the ginger water hot but not boiling, since each time the towel is dipped heat will be lost. Keep the pan covered when not dipping the towel, or heat it intermittently.

Apply the hot towel to the affected area. If it is too hot, let it cool in the air before applying it to the skin. A thin dry towel may be used between the skin and the hot towels until the hot towels can be applied directly to the skin without discomfort. Cover the hot towel with a dry bath towel to keep the area being treated warm. Use two towels, and apply newly dipped towels every few minutes for 10 to 25 minutes. When changing towels, lift the dry bath towel and the previously applied towel off the skin and replace with a newly dipped towel and the same dry bath towel. This keeps the area as warm as possible with the least amount of cooling between towels. Stop when the area has turned red, or when the pain is gone. Ginger compresses applied to the kidney area are very relaxing.

—Albi (Taro Potato) Plaster—

The albi plaster is often used following a ginger compress. It is useful for relieving pain and helping to remove excess toxins from the body. Like the ginger compress, an albi plaster is quite powerful and caution is needed in certain conditions. It may be used with confidence on the body if cancer or other serious illness is not present. Consult home remedy books or a trained macrobiotic counselor before using an albi plaster on a person with cancer or if you wish to use an albi plaster on a person's head. Albi (taro potato) may be found in Asian markets, some natural food stores, and some mail order catalogs. Powdered albi is available but fresh albi is preferred.

Choose a light-colored (more white) albi that is small and fresh. Peel the albi and discard the skin. Grate the albi using a Japanese grater. Grate enough fresh ginger to equal 10 percent of the amount of albi and mix together. (If the plaster causes itchiness, reduce the amount of ginger next time.) Add unbleached white flour until the mixture is the consistency of an earlobe, like thick dough or paste. Spread the mixture on a cotton cloth—flannel works well—to a depth of one-half inch, and apply the paste side directly on the area being treated. Secure with a gauze bandage if necessary. Leave the albi on for up to 4 hours. Discard after removing and do not reuse, as it will be full of toxins.

—Tofu Plaster—

The main uses of a tofu plaster are to relieve head pain; to reduce very high fevers; to provide cooling relief to overly heated areas (such as in inflammations) of the body or head; and in emergency cases of internal bleeding where medical help is unavailable. Any kind of tofu may be used. Squeeze the excess water out of a block of tofu and then mash well. Beat the tofu to remove lumps, and add 1 tablespoon peeled and grated ginger per 8 ounces of tofu. Next, add enough unbleached white flour to make the mixture sticky. Apply directly to the area being treated, about 3/4-inch thick, and secure with a bandage. Leave on for 2 to 3 hours or until the plaster turns yellow or becomes hot. In cases of fever, apply to the forehead. Change more often for high fevers or when used on the chest. Discard the plaster after using it.

—Salt Bath—

Herman Aihara popularized the salt bath for improving the overall condition of the kidneys; correcting mineral imbalances in the body; and for relieving pain, insomnia, worry, or other stress. The optimum salt bath contains 1 to 2 percent salt. Less than 1 percent is not effective and more than 2 percent is too strong. Any kind of salt may be used; use the cheapest salt available. One pound of salt in 12 gallons of bath water makes a 1 percent salt solution. Fill a tub using an empty gallon container and mark the tub at the height of 12 gallons. (Next time just fill the tub to the mark.) Any comfortable temperature of water may be used. Simply sit in the water for 20 minutes or longer. A person with a weak heart should avoid extremely hot water. He or she should stay in the tub only 5 to 10 minutes at the most and get out immediately if the heart starts beating faster or there is any discomfort in the chest area.

—Daikon Hip Bath—

The daikon hip, or sitz, bath is useful for bladder inflammation, menstrual cramps, ovarian and uterine problems, and many other female disorders, as well as for postpartum care of the mother. It also is useful for skin problems, for eliminating excess fat or oil from the body, and for anal pain.

Daikon root is sold in many stores, but often the greens are discarded. Ask the produce manager if you can have or buy the greens. Natural food stores leave the greens on the daikon. Some mail-order suppliers sell bags of dried daikon leaves ready for use. Hang fresh greens in the shade to dry until they are brown and somewhat brittle—about four to seven days. Put the dried greens from 7 daikons (about 8 cups) in a pan with 15 cups of water, bring to a boil, and simmer for 30 to 60 minutes. The water will turn dark brown in color. Add ¼ cup of any kind of salt and turn off the heat. Strain and let the water sit for 5 to 10 minutes. Pour the liquid into a small tub (big enough to sit in) and add enough hot water so that the bather's hip bones are covered. The feet and hands remain out of the daikon water. Cover the upper body and legs with a large towel or blanket to stay warm and to induce sweating. Stay in the bath for 15 to 20 minutes or until the hips become red or very hot, or the bather wishes to stop sweating. After drying off, keep the hip area warm. It is best to take the bath immediately before going to sleep. If it is taken during the day, wait at least one hour after eating and rest for at least 30 minutes after bathing before becoming active. Drink some sho-ban tea if overly tired.

—Bancha Tea—

Bancha tea is the basic macrobiotic beverage. It is useful as a daily beverage or for any disorder involving weakness or poor blood circulation. It also helps satisfy cravings for sweet foods after a meal. Bancha tea is made from twigs or stems (about 60 percent) and leaves (about 40 percent of the tea plant). It is called kukicha twig beverage if made from 100 percent twigs or stems. Place ¼ cup bancha tea (twigs, or twigs and leaves) in 4 cups water and bring to boil. Simmer for 20 minutes. Strain and serve hot.

—Sho-ban Tea—

Sho-ban tea is useful for fatigue, anemia, and any yin disorder, overly acidic condition, or weakness. It helps strengthen the blood and promotes good blood circulation. Place 1 teaspoon soy sauce in a cup and add ⅔ cup boiling bancha tea. Drink hot. Decrease the proportion of soy sauce to tea if a weaker tea is desired.

—Umesho Bancha Tea—

This tea is useful for digestive disorders, fatigue, and all cancers. It also helps improve blood circulation, regulate the heart rate, and strengthen the reproductive organs after the delivery of a baby. Umeboshi plums are plums pickled with salt and beefsteak leaves. They are available from natural food stores or mail order suppliers. Bring ½ umeboshi plum (pit removed) and ⅔ cup already prepared bancha tea to a boil and simmer for 5 minutes. Grate enough fresh ginger to yield ¼ teaspoon ginger juice after the ginger is squeezed. Place the ginger juice and ½ teaspoon soy sauce in a cup and add the umeboshi bancha tea. Drink hot.

—Umesho Kuzu Tea—

This tea is useful for diarrhea, upset stomach, and a lack of appetite. Kuzu, a starch extracted from the root of a wild Japanese plant, has a strong contracting power. It is available from natural food stores and mail order suppliers. For adults, break an umeboshi plum into several pieces, add 1½ cups water, and bring to a boil. Dissolve 1 tablespoon kuzu in 3 tablespoons cold water and add to pot. Simmer, stirring constantly until the liquid becomes clear. Add 1 teaspoon soy sauce and bring to boil. As soon as it boils remove from heat and add about 7 drops of juice squeezed from freshly grated ginger. Drink immediately. For kids, increase the kuzu to 1½ tablespoons and decrease the soy sauce to ½ teaspoon.

—Kuzu Bancha Tea—

Kuzu bancha tea is another useful tea for the intestines. Dissolve 1 teaspoon kuzu in 1 tablespoon cold water in a cup. Add 1 cup boiling bancha tea and a pinch of sea salt. Drink as soon as the kuzu turns from a milky color to clear.

—Lotus Root Tea—

This is helpful for all respiratory problems, including congestion, coughs, and sinus problems. Fresh lotus root is best, but dried or powdered lotus root may be used if necessary. For adults, grate about ½ cup lotus root, place in cheesecloth, and squeeze out the juice. For 3 tablespoons of lotus root juice, add 1 teaspoon ginger juice, a pinch of sea salt, and 1 cup water. Boil slightly and drink hot or warm. For children, use 1 tablespoon lotus root juice, 2 to 3 drops ginger juice, a pinch of sea salt, and ½ cup water. To use dried or powdered lotus root, follow the directions on the package to make 1 cup (½ cup for children) of tea. Then, add ginger and a pinch of sea salt as above.

Other Factors in Health

Eating well and wisely is only one of the factors that affect health. Indeed, everything we eat, breathe, see, hear, touch, smell, feel, think, and experience influences health. And because everything is connected and related, each factor affects all the others. For example, a stressful situation often affects your overall attitude and ability to get a good night's sleep, causing you to be cranky with loved ones or friends. Thus, learning to give proper emphasis to each area of your life helps you move toward a more balanced condition. Similarly, being unbalanced in any area tends to be unsettling in general. Different factors affect people differently, depending upon their condition and personality. This chapter discusses a few factors that tend to be most important for many people.

Attitude: People who are happy and positive about life tend to have an easier time with the healing process. People who are fearful or negative tend to have a harder time. There are two types of fear: normal fear, when one is in danger, and abnormal fear, when one is fearful of life itself. Abnormal fear, especially the fear that one cannot heal, is the greatest destroyer of human health. It leads to negative thinking. Health is positive thinking. Healing is the process of going from negative thinking (I can't) to positive thinking (I can). Abnormal fear can affect the immune system. Strong abnormal fear leads to depressed T-cells, which leads to a weakened immune system, which leads to greater sickness, which in turn leads to yet greater fear. One of the greatest benefits of macrobiotic thinking is the belief that everything can and will change. One can reverse the cycle of abnormal fear, repair the immune system, and thus achieve greater health and less abnormal fear. Love is the greatest benefactor to health, and the greatest expression of love is to live within the natural order of life. One who can do this completely will be healthy and will be able to overcome all abnormal fear of life.

Adaptability: Being able to adapt to change is very important for a healthy life. Sickness can be viewed as stagnation or blockage, either physical or mental. The remedy is to create movement. Ohsawa suggested that people learn to be adaptable. His ideas were to learn to cook whole foods, to raise or be around kids, or to visit a totally different culture. Long-time macrobiotic people sometimes lose adaptability, especially if their practice of macrobiotics is to follow a rigid set of rules. Following lists and guidelines from others is needed at first, but at some point one must create one's own lists and guidelines.

Breathing: Breathing happens without any conscious effort, but it is so important to health that learning to breathe fully and deeply can be very beneficial. There are two main functions of breathing. Inhaling brings oxygen into the body. If the breathing is complete and full, the air is of good quality, and if there are no blockages in the body, the cells get the oxygen they need. Exhaling removes about 70 percent of the body's wastes and contributes greatly to well-being. If the quality of the air you breathe is poor, you might consider an air purifier for your home. Also, the more house plants you have the better.

Sunshine: Sunshine lifts the spirits. Today, there are warnings about spending too much time in the sun without a sun block to protect the skin. However, if the body's healing power is reasonably strong, one can enjoy moderate time in the sun without needless worry. For longer times in the sun some protection is needed. Natural sun blocks are available from natural food stores, and are better than other sun blocks. However, there are some indications that the active ingredients in all sun blocks may be harmful.

Environment: The quality of the surrounding environment is becoming more and more important. Breathing clean air and consuming pure water is particularly important. Natural unpolluted spring water is best, but is getting harder to find. Well-water is another good source if not contaminated. Water filters also work well.

An increasing number of natural products are available, including natural foods, natural clothing, natural insect repellents, and natural cosmetics. One might first pay attention to the things closest to the body, such as clothing and cosmetics, and to the places one spends a substantial amount of time, such as the bed. Natural products are those substances that exist in nature and are as close to the way nature provides them as possible. For example, cotton, wool, and silk are natural fibers that promote health. Polyester is a manufactured product that is not natural and wearing it does not promote health.

In my experience, people who change to a macrobiotic approach first become more sensitive to environmental pollutants, and later gain strength for dealing with them. It is best to eliminate as many pollutants as possible. Houses and modern-day workplaces often do more to hinder health than promote it.

Social support: Health depends partly on friendship because a friend shares life's stresses and joys, and supports one's decisions. This reduces one's stress and improves one's self-esteem. The number of true friends a person has can be an indicator of her or his level of health. Friendships, like all relationships, require give and take, but some take more time and effort than others. Relationships that create excess stress can be damaging to health and may need some time and space. Sometimes improved health can lead to an improved friendship.

People who follow a macrobiotic approach need not lose their friends who do not follow such an approach; nor need they stop going to parties. If one cannot avoid sugary foods or meat, one can eat a small amount and chew it well. Or simply saying "My condition does not allow me to eat these foods," is a response that should not make other people uncomfortable about what they are eating.

Making new friends who are making similar changes in their lives can be rewarding. A note on a message board at a local natural food store, announcing a macrobiotic potluck or merely stating one's interest in finding other macrobiotic people, is one way. There are also macrobiotic gatherings such as the French Meadows Summer Camp.

Stress: Stress has become a large factor in most people's health. Stresses at work, financial concerns, and family matters can be energy drainers. Dealing with unusual stress such as the death of a loved one or the loss of a job only adds to the amount of energy it takes to deal with everyday stress. Being open and honest and dealing with as much pain as possible when the loss occurs is best. As overall health improves, one's ability to deal with everyday stress and unusual stress also increases. Stress is acid-forming, so more alkaline-forming food and activities can be helpful.

A relative of stress is overworry. Macrobiotic people often worry too much about whether or not to eat a certain food. The worry can be more detrimental than the food; eat it and be happy, or don't eat it and don't worry about it.

Electronics: Advances in technology make life more simple and enjoyable in some ways but the cost in terms of health is oftentimes high. For example, computers can speed work, but even moderate use can cause headaches and other symptoms, even if you have a good diet, frequent breaks, radiation shields, etc.

Television can consume too much time. People have reported that frequent headaches disappear when they stop watching television or sleeping near a clock radio. Microwaves "heat" food by making the molecules move in a chaotic and unnatural manner. The effect on a person's health may be negative and caution is advised.

While there is no reason to avoid all machines, a person who is sick—especially if the sickness is stubborn and hard to cure—should try to determine whether some machine may be a cause of or a contributor to the discomfort. Books on applied kinesiology and biofeedback can provide further information.

Religious values: All religions and religious practices fit well with a macrobiotic lifestyle. In other words, a macrobiotic approach can be used by members of any religion. The macrobiotic viewpoint is that everyone is a part of Oneness (God), and that a positive relationship with one's Creator, God, Oneness, Infinity (or whatever the name) is very important. Knowing who one is, where one comes from, and where one is going spiritually provides tremendous healing power.

Sleep: Good sleep is necessary for good health, and it is a sign of good health. Having trouble falling asleep or not sleeping deeply through the night is a signal something is wrong, such as a poor diet or strong emotional stress, and action must be taken. It is important that the bed be comfortable and made of natural products; then, after major excesses have been discharged, sleep will be good and deep.

The general macrobiotic recommendation is not to eat before going to bed—some say for up to three hours. The amount of sleep one needs will most likely vary as one's health changes. Too much sleep can be more tiring than too little sleep. In any event, it is normal to wake up refreshed and ready to meet the challenges of the day. If one doesn't, this is a signal that one's condition is not the best.

Sex: The macrobiotic view is that sex is a unification of opposites, yin and yang, and thus an expression of the natural order of life. Many macrobiotic people report better sex and an increased sexual appetite once their body's natural health is restored. I have heard of some couples who were previously unable to conceive who have conceived and delivered healthy babies after a switch to a macrobiotic dietary approach.

Movement: Activity is necessary to use food fully. In fact, a lack of exercise is one of the main reasons why some long-time macrobiotic followers feel fatigued. There are many forms of exercise, including weight lifting, jogging, hiking, calisthenics, gardening, yoga, aikido, and house cleaning. People with cancer or other serious illness should take milder forms of exercise, such as non-strenuous gardening and walking. A person who is at all uncertain about exercising should check with a health care advisor before beginning any exercise program, especially a strenuous one.

Appendix

Toward Macrobiotic Living

There are as many ways to learn macrobiotics as there are people. In talking to people over the years, I have heard of many different approaches. Some want to change quickly, others take their time and ease into it more gradually. Some want to learn all they can about macrobiotic principles and increase their understanding and enjoyment of life as much as possible using those principles. Others are content to follow a macrobiotic dietary approach and enjoy more limited benefits. Some will be moved to begin a macrobiotic lifestyle the minute they read or hear a fair presentation of it. Others wait until they have cancer or some other major disease. Some people love the idea of being self-reliant. Others will never feel comfortable being in charge or control of their own destiny—they are happier paying for and accepting the advice of others, be they macrobiotic counselors, alternative health advisors, or medical doctors.

In my opinion, the biggest mistake in macrobiotic education is giving information to people rather than teaching them how to think. From an early age, most people are taught to believe others rather than to trust in their own judgment. Giving knowledge in the form of lists of things to eat or do and things not to eat or do is fine for a beginning but in the long run creates slaves instead of free persons who can think for themselves. It is your life and it depends on your decisions. Thus, improving your judgment is most important.

This does not mean that you shouldn't accept the advice and help of others when it is needed. A macrobiotic lifestyle is learning from life. It includes doctors and other professionals, books and nature, family and friends, successes and failures, sickness and health, and on and on. Each person is a part of the totality of life and experiences only a part of life; life is bigger than any one person's perception of it. It is bigger than any theory of it, including macrobiotics.

Macrobiotics is a study of life—the natural laws of change. But like any expression of life, it is only a partial picture. Using a macrobiotic approach to life as a tool, you can begin to see more of the total picture—it becomes clearer, more focused. The whole picture is there all the time but your view of it changes as your ability to focus—your judgment—increases or decreases. More clarity comes from increasing your judgment, which comes from a greater understanding of the natural laws of change, which in turn comes from eating well and living in harmony with the natural order of life. Blindly following a prescribed set of rules is not the goal of macrobiotics. Instead, the goal is to live a happy and healthy life in which you freely make your own decisions and gladly accept the consequences of those decisions. You always will need books and other people to give you guidance and to answer your questions, but after a while you need to begin to rely more on your own judgment and to answer your own questions.

The suggestions offered here are based on my experience in talking with many people over many years about beginning a macrobiotic approach to life. There are many roads to the final destination, but the idea and willingness to begin must come from you. How to begin and how to travel is outlined here, but the decision to travel, the speed at which you go, and the direction are totally up to you.

- Be prepared to change. Macrobiotics is a philosophy of change that leads to the oneness or unification of all things. Many thinkers in many centuries have taught change. When you begin macrobiotic practice, you will change. You can control the rate of change by the rate at which you make dietary and lifestyle changes. If you are inspired to change all at once, go for it—just do it. If you prefer a slower transition, this is okay also. In either case, being prepared for and open to change will ease the transition. A healthy life includes both constancy and change.

- Gain a working knowledge of the concepts and principles behind macrobiotics. Reread and study the chapters on yin and yang and healing as you proceed. You will find that your understanding of the principles changes, even though they are constant.
- Be realistic about the results that can be reasonably expected. In order to gain a wider appeal for macrobiotics, some authors have made it sound very easy to gain fantastic results. This book attempts to provide enough information so that there are not many unexpected changes. Many people drop out of macrobiotic living because of unrealistic expectations.
- Develop a plan. There are many books on how to develop a plan for changing different kinds of behavior. While these may be helpful, people often spend more time in planning than in doing. Still, there are several areas or plan development that are worth considering.

  - Breaking the large overall goal up into smaller ones can be useful to get started. Set attainable goals, a time limit for reaching the goal, and a reward that you will give yourself for making progress toward reaching the goal.
  - Knowing yourself, your strengths, weaknesses, and present condition allows you to honestly evaluate your chances of success and helps you set reasonable goals.
  - Knowing the resources available to help you reach your goals is probably the most helpful. For example, in addition to your own personal resources, there are macrobiotic counselors, support persons, study centers, camps and conferences, books, magazines, directories, natural food stores, mail order suppliers, family, friends, and so on. (See the Resources section.) Having a support person to whom you report your progress can

be helpful. Knowing others who are working toward similar goals can be very valuable; you can share experiences and understandings.

- Establish helpful everyday habits. Here is a list of habits that can be valuable.

– Exercise. At the very least, give yourself five to ten minutes a day of stretching and organized movement that includes breathing deeply.
– Chew well. One of the best exercises is chewing food. If you feel sick, try to double the amount of chewing for each mouthful.
– Reflect. Give yourself five to ten minutes time each day to reflect on the day, relationships, and yin and yang. And listen to nature each day as much as possible.
– Eat sensibly. Eat a grain-centered diet without being overly rigid or fanatic (unless your condition demands it). Your daily diet is most important; an occasional deviation can be refreshing and easily tolerated.
– Write. Write in a personal journal every day. Writing about what happened and your reactions to what happened is enough. Or write to family and friends about your experiences.
– Read. Reading inspiring and supportive literature, even one page a day, is very helpful.
– Check-up. Pay attention to your condition every day, especially after the initial discharge period, by checking your urine, feces, and body for warning signals of imbalance.
– Create. Choose a hobby that allows you to express yourself, such as playing music, writing poetry or novels, painting, drawing, acting, and so on. Or, be creative in thinking of ways to help others or yourself.
– Contemplate oneness. For at least one moment every day stop and view life from the perspective of oneness. From

this view, no person is better than any other person, or any other thing for that matter. Every one and every thing is connected. Most people spend too much time looking at what separates us rather than at what unites us.

These are some ideas for developing a macrobiotic approach to living. I sincerely hope that you will find these suggestions useful and that you will develop your own lists and your own plan. You can and should be the director of your own life. Always ask questions and answer them yourself to gain a deeper understanding of oneness. This is the macrobiotic way.

As your natural judging ability and instinct increases, you will be able to live a more healthy and happy life. Then, you can go beyond beginning macrobiotics and become eternally peaceful and infinitely free. It is the understanding of the natural order of all things, the oneness of all things, and the changeability of all things that allows you to live a life that is truly happy, healthy, and free.

Exercises in Distinguishing Yin and Yang

Learning to use yin and yang is like learning a new language or musical instrument—it takes time and practice. In order to learn a new language you have to practice with that language. Any amount of working knowledge you obtain is useful and allows you to learn more. At some point, yin and yang, just like a new language, becomes instinctive and you no longer have to think about the elementary concepts in order to use them in your daily life.

Practicing every day, even though the time may be brief, is better than the same amount of total time spent all at once. It is helpful to work with yin and yang each day for at least 10 minutes. Many people who try to learn yin and yang too quickly and all at once become frustrated and confused. A working knowledge of yin and yang only comes with daily practice over a period of time. This time can be spent studying this or other books and magazine articles on yin and yang, or practicing discriminating between yin and yang among common objects or within your own body.

Any of the following exercises can increase your working knowledge of yin and yang. During the first year of macrobiotic practice reread these suggestions at least once a month. After the first year reread the chapter on macrobiotic yin and yang from time to time. You'll be surprised how your understanding deepens over time. As you practice with the ideas that follow, refer to the principles and charts as needed. These exercises can be used in any order.

- Go to the store and pick any vegetable or fruit to study. For example, pick up any two red delicious apples. In terms of size, the smaller one is more yang (less yin) and the larger one is more yin. In terms of color, the darker one is more yang (less yin) and the lighter one is more yin. After you have evaluated the apples for as many characteristics as possible, find the two most similar apples and the two farthest apart in yin and yang qualities. Each time you visit the store, follow the same process with another vegetable or fruit.

- While at the store, choose two different vegetables or two different fruits and evaluate their yin or yang characteristics. The first few times choose similar vegetables such as carrots and parsnips or kale and collards. Compare different varieties of the same fruit such as red delicious apples and Granny Smith apples. Later, compare carrots and kale or apples and oranges in terms of yin and yang.

- Using the procedures in exercise 1, buy an amount of carrots that are more yin and the same amount of carrots that are more yang (less yin). Using the same cutting and cooking method, and ideally the same kind of pan and heat, compare the yin carrots and the yang carrots in terms of their effect on you. Did they cook the same or differently? The more differences and similarities you can determine the better.

- Using the same manner of preparation and cooking method, compare the effects of similar vegetables such as carrots and parsnips and then very different vegetables such as carrots and leafy greens. People's reactions vary. One person may find that buckwheat has a more yin (cooling) effect, and another may feel a more yang (warming) effect. Both reactions are valid and demonstrate the variable nature of yin and yang. Similarly, you may not always notice a difference between similar vegetables.

- Compare organic vegetables and non-organic vegetables in terms of yin and yang characteristics, taste, and vitality; that is, the energy you get from eating each. The difference can be quite subtle or indistinguishable. For example, I find that organic ones taste better and seem to have more vitality, giving me more energy once eaten.

- Study the effect different cooking preparations have on you. Is there a difference between vegetables cooked with salt and vegetables with sweetener added? Boiled carrots versus baked carrots are very different in their appearance and effect. Just by paying attention to the differences, you will become very familiar with yin and yang.

- If you are cooking on an electric stove or using a microwave, find a way to cook over gas or wood heat for at least a month and compare the difference in how you feel. If you are fatigued much of the time, a change to gas or wood heat can have a positive effect. If you have a sensitivity to natural gas, check your appliances for leaks and correct any found.

- Look in the mirror daily and honestly evaluate your condition. Pay most attention to the factors that change the most. Is your face more red (yang) or more pale (yin) in color? Do you have any puffiness or swelling (yin) anywhere? Evaluate the condition of your eliminations. Are they more yin or more yang? What does this tell you about the food you ate yesterday?

- Pay attention to how your emotions and mental conditions change, both due to seasonal changes and to daily dietary changes. Ask yourself how you feel every day. After some time these evaluations become automatic.

- Compare yourself with family members or friends. Decide who is most yin and most yang in terms of height, weight, and other physical conditions. Compare emotional and mental conditions also. If you know someone else learning yin and yang compare your evaluations. The store or the office is a good place to look at people in terms of yin or yang. It does not take long to tell the difference between meat eaters and vegetarians, for example. Another fun thing to do is to look at people in the store and what's in their shopping baskets. After a while you only have to look at one to know the other.
- Compare other books or magazine articles on yin and yang and diagnosis with this book. If your experience indicates a different yin or yang order, change the charts accordingly.
- Make up your own questions and find the answers yourself. This is most important for your continued development.

If you are making big changes in your diet, your body will be throwing out stored toxins. Evaluations of the effects of certain foods or cooking methods may need to wait until your body has rid itself of these toxins.

Don't worry if yin and yang seems difficult to learn—a change in diet is more important at first. Taking your time and learning every step completely will give you a deeper understanding and greater working knowledge of yin and yang in particular and of life in general.

Using Macrobiotic Principles: Friends and Enemies

Those who have friends, have enemies. Ohsawa's macrobiotic theory is practical for daily living. It is based on the idea that it is possible to change anything to its opposite—sickness to health, sadness to happiness, war to peace, enslavement to freedom, hate to love, separation to unification. Here is a simplified look at the possibilities of changing enemies to friends using macrobiotic principles. Much more could be written about each of these concepts and extensive study of Ohsawa's original works is highly recommended.

The Order of the Universe: We start with the order of the universe because it is Ohsawa's explanation of how we got here—our "physical" transformation from the infinite to individuals. This process occurs in seven stages or worlds. What is important to understand is that each world creates and nourishes the next world and thus all worlds below it. The infinite world creates and nourishes the world of polarity. Together they create and nourish the world of vibration. These three create and nourish the pre-atomic world, the world of elements, then the plant world, and finally the animal world, of which we are a part.

We are nourished by vegetal foods; elements including air, sunshine, and water; pre-atomic particles; vibration or energy; polarity or opposition; and the Infinite itself. Ohsawa taught that the more we align ourselves with this natural order, the healthier we become and the more we are able to resolve any conflict.

Here, then, is our first step in changing enemies to friends. Eat whole grain and vegetable foods in as unaltered a form as possible. Pay attention to the quality of air and water, and filter these if needed. Avoid chemicalized foods and those with artificial additives or preservatives because these foods lead us away from the natural order.

The Seven Laws: The seven laws of the order of the universe and the twelve theorems of the unique principle are Ohsawa's teachings to be used like a compass in making daily decisions. Here is a look at the seven laws from the perspective of enemies and friends.

"What has a beginning has an end." The conflict began at some time; it will end at some time. Generally, conflicts that develop quickly resolve more quickly and those that develop over a longer period of time take longer to resolve.

"What has a front has a back." If a friend is considered as a "front," that friend also can become an enemy (a "back"). "The bigger the front, the bigger the back." The greater the friend, the greater the potential enemy. Conversely, the greater the enemy, the greater the potential friend.

"There is nothing identical." Every situation/conflict is different and constantly changing. The trick is to learn how to turn the situation in the desired direction—toward resolution.

"Every antagonism is complementary." And, "yin (enemies) and yang (friends) are the classifications of all polarization (relationships). They are antagonistic and complementary." A perceived enemy is seen as antagonistic to us. Yet, the enemy also is complementary—a necessary part to complete the whole. We know what it means to have friends because we know what it means to have enemies. Both are necessary. Enemies provide us with the opportunity to learn, to grow, and to elevate our judgment.

"Yin and yang are the two arms of One (Infinite)." Both friends and enemies are part of One Infinite. The Infinite accepts both and so should we. Truly understanding these last two laws can lead to resolution of any conflict.

The Twelve Theorems: Ohsawa's twelve theorems of the unifying principle use the terms "yin" and yang." However, any pair of opposites can be substituted for yin and yang for greater understanding. Here are the twelve theorems using enmity or enemies and friendship or friends in place of yin and yang as applied to relationships.

1. Enmity and friendship are two poles that enter into play when the infinite expansion manifests itself at the point of division. Enemies and friends are manifestations of the Infinite.

2. Enmity and friendship are produced continually by the tran-

scendental expansion. Transcendental expansion is another name for the Infinite, beyond our experience but not beyond our intuitive knowledge.

3. Enmity is centrifugal. Friendship is centripetal. Enmity and friendship produce energy. We keep enemies at bay. We hold friends close. Enemies keep us on our toes.

4. Enmity attracts friendship. Friendship attracts enmity. Everything is attracted to its opposite. Another way to look at this theorem is that without an enemy, life would be boring. We would become complacent and seek an enemy for contrast and excitement.

5. Enmity and friendship combined in variable proportion comprise all relationships. There is a force of attraction toward friendship and of repulsion toward enmity in every relationship.

6. All relationships are ephemeral, being infinitely complex and constantly changing enmity and friendship components. Every relationship is without rest. Friends become enemies and enemies become friends. The real question is the direction the relationship is heading.

7. No one is totally an enemy or totally a friend, even in the most apparently simple relationship. Every relationship contains a polarity at all times. There will be arguments, disagreements, or conflicts of varying degrees in every relationship. Realizing this can lead to less worry when conflicts occur.

8. No relationship is neutral. Enmity and friendship is in excess in every case. We perceive others as enemies or friends at every moment, even though at any moment a friend can become an enemy or an enemy can become a friend.

9. The force of attraction is proportional to the difference of the enmity and friendship components. The greater the perceived enemy the more of our attention that enemy receives.

10. Enmity repels enmity and friendship repels friendship. The force of repulsion or attraction is inversely proportional to the degree of enmity or friendship. With a good friend there is more opportunity and likelihood for disagreement or conflict because we are around them more often than a marginal friend.

11. Over time and within the space of the finite world, enmity produces friendship, and friendship produces enmity. Every relationship will change sooner or later.

12. Every physical body is more friendly at its center and more adversarial toward its surface. The heart is more loving and the limbs more ready for a fight. It is said of some men, "he wears his emotions on his sleeves." Centering oneself in any conflict is a way to turn the direction of that conflict toward resolution.

Stages of Judgment: The stages of judgment are Ohsawa's explanation of our "spiritual" transformation from birth to reunification with the Infinite. What is the first thing we did when we were born? Breathe? Cry? Eat? In the womb, every thing is provided—all our needs are met automatically. Our consciousness develops in a mechanical way.

Then, everything changes. Suddenly, we're outside and separated. We have to adapt. We become aware of our senses. This is the beginning of sensorial judgment or consciousness. Next we begin to discriminate between what we like and dislike. This is sentimental or emotional judgment. Our ability to reason or intellectual judgment comes next followed by our ability to distinguish ourselves from others. We become aware of family, community, and friends. This is social judgment. We then begin to judge what is good and bad, or right and wrong, often from a doctrinal perspective. This is ideological judgment. Each of us develops these six stages to some degree. The seventh stage is supreme judgment or unconditional love.

One way to change enemies to friends is to work on elevating our judgment by understanding, and then developing, each judgment. It is growth in each individual stage of judgment that leads to elevation of judgment to higher levels within each stage and finally to supreme judgment. In any conflict, if one person can elevate her or his consciousness or judgment, resolution is possible.

When someone hits us, if we hit back we are responding at the same level. This is mechanical judgment. On the sensory level, we see that our enemies are different from us. Our enemies see us as different from them. On the sentimental level, we dislike them and they dislike us. We would be more comfortable without them around us and vice versa. On the intellectual level we justify our reasons for the conflict. On the social level, we come up with moral, and sometimes economic, reasons for the conflict. On the ideological level, we believe we are right and they believe they are right.

Even if we understand all of this, the conflict continues. Why? The conflict continues because both sides are at the same level at every stage of judgment. As long as we feel that we are different from them, better than them, and right or justified in our actions, and they feel exactly the same way, resolution is next to impossible. There is only one real solution and that comes from recognizing the real underlying cause of this, and of every, conflict.

The underlying cause of every conflict is what makes us human in the first place, separation. It is the first thing we feel when we enter this world at birth. It is why we breathe. It is why we eat. It is why we cry. Our conscious or spiritual life is our journey to reconnect with the Infinite. If and when we do this, we begin to understand that there are no differences – we are they and they are we. Neither is better or worse. Neither is right or wrong. There simply is no need for conflict—the Infinite loves us all equally and unconditionally.

Elevation of consciousness to such a state is extremely difficult. Being human, we carry all the stages of judgment with us all the time. The six "lower" stages dominate our thinking and emotions most of the time. Glimpses of the supreme judgment or unconditional love are possible during moments of grace or during periods of deep meditation or contemplation.

Summary: Here are some ideas to help elevate consciousness and to help resolve individual conflicts in daily living.

1. Strengthen yourself by eating primarily unaltered whole grains and fresh vegetable foods and by working hard. By so doing, one's mechanical judgment becomes clear and precise, leading to greater health. Through greater health, a glimpse of supreme judgment is revealed.

2. To elevate consciousness, take little and give much. Here is a slightly edited quote from Lao Tsu's Tao Te Ching, "Nature just gives. One who gives always accomplishes everything because such a person is Nature."

3. In any conflict, realize that both parties are at fault. Spend whatever time it takes to fully understand your part. What you dislike is your responsibility and is changeable.

4. Study and understand the order of the universe and other macrobiotic teachings. Learn to unify (change the direction of) all apparent opposites.

5. Keep busy by doing hard physical work and by doing things for others. Giving to others is a way to improve your spiritual power. Ohsawa encourages us to emulate the biological law: from one grain comes ten thousand grains.

6. Realize that it is easier to change your behavior than someone else's. To change someone else you must be a very great person spiritually.

7. Reduce your ego desires for transitory things. Do not attach yourself to the finite/ephemeral world, as everything in it is transitory and will end sooner or later. Rather, attach yourself to the Infinite. Give up things you like so others can have more.

8. Understand that every one has the capacity for supreme judgment or love but that it is often eclipsed or veiled by sensorial or sentimental love. Here is a quote from Herman Aihara's *Learning from Salmon*: "Only when we humbly admit our own smallness, exclusively, sensorial, and sentimental love can we admit and accept the smallness of others. Therefore we are able to embrace them. This is supreme love."

Once we truly understand and learn to use these principles in our daily lives, all conflicts are resolved and all enemies become friends.

Ohsawa's Order of the Universe

Stages of Life	Orbit/World	Beginning of	Antagonisms and Complementaries
Infinite Expansion	7. Infinity, God Oneness	The world that has no beginning or end	There is no specialization: all analytical, mechanical, and statistical science is invalid in the infinite world.
Inorganic	6. Polarization	The foundation of the relative world	The polarization of the Infinite into yin (expansion) and yang (contraction)—the origin of magnetism.
	5. Vibration	The production of energy and origin of electricity	Visible and invisible radiation, hot and cold rays, dynamic and stimulating rays (yellow, orange, red) and static and calming rays (green, blue, indigo, violet), infrared and ultra-violet radiation.
	4. Pre-atomic particles	Electrons, protons, and all sub-atomic particles	Centrifugal and centripetal force, solid and gaseous.
	3. Elements	Atoms, stars, and millions of solar systems	Mountain and river, land and sea, air and earth, polar and tropical regions, hot and cold, day and night, surface and center of Earth.
Organic	2. Vegetable	Viruses, bacteria, and all plants	Grass and tree, trunk and branch, branch and leaf, flower and seed (or fruit), cell and organ, germ and soma cells.
	1. Animal	All animals, including human beings	White and red corpuscles, bone and flesh, man and woman, governors and governed, worker and capitalist, work and rest, love and hate, war and peace, sickness and health, life and death.

Excerpted and adapted from George Ohsawa's *Essential Ohsawa* by Carl Ferré; *www.ohsawamacrobiotics.com.*

Ohsawa's Seven Laws and Twelve Theorems

The Seven Laws of the Order of the Universe

1. What has a beginning has an end.
2. What has a front has a back.
3. There is nothing identical.
4. The bigger the front, the bigger the back.
5. Every antagonism is complementary.
6. Yin and Yang are the classifications of all polarization. They are antagonistic and complementary.
7. Yin and Yang are the two arms of One (Infinite).

The Twelve Theorems of the Unique Principle

1. Yin-Yang are two poles which enter into play when the infinite expansion manifests itself at the point of bifurcation.
2. Yin-Yang are produced continually by the transcendental expansion.
3. Yin is centrifugal. Yang is centripetal. Yin and Yang produce energy.
4. Yin attracts Yang. Yang attracts Yin.
5. Yin and Yang combined in variable proportion produce all phenomena.
6. All phenomena are ephemeral, being of infinitely complex constitutions and constantly changing Yin and Yang components. Everything is without rest.
7. Nothing is totally Yin or totally Yang, even in the most apparently simple phenomenon. Everything contains a polarity at every stage of its composition.
8. Nothing is neutral. Yin or Yang is in excess in every case.
9. The force of attraction is proportional to the difference of the Yin and Yang components.
10. Yin repels Yin and Yang repels Yang. The repulsion is inversely proportional to the difference of the Yin and Yang forces.
11. With time and space, Yin produces Yang, and Yang produces Yin.
12. Every physical body is Yang at its center and Yin toward surface.

The seven laws and twelve theorems as written by Ohsawa in the 1962 French edition of *The Atomic Era and the Philosophy of the Far East* and as translated by Michael and Maria Chen.

Ohsawa's Seven Stages Of Judgment

Stages	Learning	Love	Profession	Eating and Drinking
1. Physical or Mechanical	Instinctive or unconscious reflexes	Instinctive, appetite, hunger	One who sells one's life (working slave, salaried employee)	Guided only by hunger or thirst
2. Sensorial	Dance, gymnastics, conditioned reflexes	Erotic, seeking physical comfort and sensual pleasure	Wholesaler of pleasure: actor, merchant, novelist, prostitute	Gourmand (greedy eater)
3. Sentimental	Literature	Emotionally universal	Wholesaler of emotions	Gourmet (connoisseur)
4. Intellectual	Science, arts	Understanding, scientific, systematic, calculating	Wholesaler of knowledge and techniques	Eating according to a theory of nutrition
5. Social	Economy, morality	Social	Organizer	Conformist—like everyone else
6. Ideological	Philosophy, religion, dialectics	Spiritual	Thinker, originator of theories	Follows dietetic or religious principle
7. Supreme, Infinite	Self-realization, illumination, tao satori	All-embracing	Happy person, fulfills all dreams throughout life	Eats and drinks anything with great pleasure

Excerpted and adapted from George Ohsawa's *Essential Ohsawa* by Carl Ferré; *www.ohsawamacrobiotics.com.*

Recommended Reading

Macrobiotic Philosophy

Ohsawa, George. *Essential Ohsawa*. Chico, CA: George Ohsawa Macrobiotic Foundation, 1994—The most comprehensive presentation of Ohsawa's philosophy. Ohsawa is the founder of modern-day macrobiotics, and *Essential Ohsawa* is a clear and understandable presentation of the scope of Ohsawa's macrobiotic thinking and spirit.

Aihara, Herman. *Basic Macrobiotics, Revised Edition*. Chico, CA: George Ohsawa Macrobiotic Foundation, 1997—Explains macrobiotics from more of a nutritional perspective than any other book and is easily accessible to Western readers. This book provides insight into the workings of a macrobiotic diet and lifestyle.

Ohsawa, George. *Zen Macrobiotics, Unabridged Edition*. Chico, CA: George Ohsawa Macrobiotic Foundation, 1995.

Ohsawa, George and Herman Aihara. *Macrobiotics: An Invitation to Health and Happiness*. Chico, CA: George Ohsawa Macrobiotic Foundation, 1971.

Ohsawa, George. *Philosophy of Oriental Medicine*. Oroville, CA: George Ohsawa Macrobiotic Foundation, 1991—Originally written in 1956 to explain macrobiotic philosophy to Dr. Albert Schweitzer, this book has been a classic of macrobiotic literature.

Ohsawa, George. *The Order of the Universe*. Chico, CA: George Ohsawa Macrobiotic Foundation, 1986.

Ohsawa, George. *Unique Principle*. Chico, CA: George Ohsawa Macrobiotic Foundation, 1973.

Macrobiotic Approach to Diet

Ferré, Julia. *Basic Macrobiotic Cooking, Twentieth Anniversary Edition*. Chico, CA: George Ohsawa Macrobiotic Foundation, 2007—The basics of cooking whole grains and fresh vegetables are clearly explained, and the many special techniques of macrobiotic cooking are presented in an easy-to-understand way.

Ferré, Julia. *French Meadows Cookbook*. Chico, CA: George Ohsawa Macrobiotic Foundation, 2008—Favorite dishes served at the annual French Meadows Summer Camp.

Aihara, Cornellia, *Calendar Cookbook*. Chico, CA: George Ohsawa Macrobiotic Foundation, 1979.

Aihara, Cornellia, ed. *The First Macrobiotic Cookbook, Revised Edition*. Chico, CA: George Ohsawa Macrobiotic Foundation, 1985.

Turner, Kristina. *Self-Healing Cookbook*. Grass Valley, CA: Earthtones Press, 1987—Accessible to both the new and the experienced cook, and integrates macrobiotics, psychology, nutrition, and a planetary view of healing.

Kushi, Aveline. *Complete Guide to Macrobiotic Cooking*. New York: Warner Books, 1985.

Colbin, Annemarie. *Food and Healing*. Tenth Anniversary Edition. New York: Ballantine Books, 1996—A comprehensive look at food and its role in the healing process. Many dietary approaches are studied and compared.

Colbin, Annemarie. *The Natural Gourmet*. New York: Ballantine Books, 1989—For those at the intermediate or advanced stage of macrobiotic understanding.

Stanchich, Lino. *Power Eating Program*. Miami, FL: Healthy Products, 1989—Useful especially for those who are not convinced that chewing food well is important.

Macrobiotic Healing

Aihara, Herman. *Acid and Alkaline, 5th edition*. Chico, CA: George Ohsawa Macrobiotic Foundation, 1986—This book is very important for a complete understanding of a macrobiotic approach to life.

Ferré, Carl. *Acid Alkaline Companion*. Chico, CA: George Ohsawa Macrobiotic Foundation, 2009.

Riviere, Francoise. *#7 Diet*. Chico, CA: George Ohsawa Macrobiotic Foundation, 2005. Detailed instructions for George Ohsawa's legendary brown rice diet.

Aihara, Cornellia and Herman Aihara with Carl Ferré. *Natural Healing from Head to Toe*. Garden City Park, NY: Avery Publishing Group, 1994—Contains an A-to-Z reference section of more than two hundred common health problems, along with numerous techniques and therapies and dietary recommendations for each disorder.

Muramoto, Noboru. *Healing Ourselves*. New York: Avon Books, 1973—One of the classics of macrobiotic literature, providing valuable insight into natural healing.

Ohsawa, George. *Practical Guide to Far Eastern Macrobiotic Medicine*. Chico, CA: George Ohsawa Macrobiotic Foundation, 1976.

Kushi, Michio and Alex Jack. *Macrobiotic Path to Total Health*. New York: Balantine Books, 2003—An in-depth guide that is useful for remedies to most disorders.

Ohsawa, George. *Cancer and the Philosophy of the Far East*. Chico, CA: George Ohsawa Macrobiotic Foundation, 1981.

Nyoiti, Sakurazawa (George Ohsawa) with William Dufty. *You Are All Sanpaku*. Secaucus, NJ: Carrol Publishing, 1965.

Kushi, Michio. *The Cancer Prevention Diet, Revised and Updated Edition*. New York: St. Martin's Griffin, 2009.

Macrobiotic Experience

Macrobiotics Today. Oroville, CA: George Ohsawa Macrobiotic Foundation, bimonthly.

Mattson, Bob. *International Macrobiotic Directory.* Oakland, CA: Bob Mattson, yearly.

Aihara, Herman. *Learning from Salmon.* Chico, CA: George Ohsawa Macrobiotic Foundation, 1980.

Heidenry, Carolyn. *Making the Transition to a Macrobiotic Diet.* Garden City Park, NY: Avery Publishing Group, 1984.

Ohsawa, George. *The Book of Judo.* Chico, CA: George Ohsawa Macrobiotic Foundation, 1990.

A current catalog of macrobiotic books is available from the George Ohsawa Macrobiotic Foundation, P. O. Box 3998, Chico, CA 95927-3998. To request a catalog or to place an order, call (530) 566-9765 or (800) 232-2372. Or, see *www.ohsawamacrobiotics.com.*

Macrobiotic Resources

Macrobiotic teachers can be found in most larger cities; there are many macrobiotic titles in the George Ohsawa Macrobiotic Foundation catalog; and macrobiotic supplies can be obtained at local natural food stores or by mail. The George Ohsawa Macrobiotic Foundation maintains a current list of centers and people who can provide further information in your area. Call 800-232-2372 or 530-566-9765 and ask for a current catalog.

Another way to learn more about macrobiotics is with a subscription to *Macrobiotics Today* magazine. In addition to informative and inspiring articles on macrobiotic subjects, *Macrobiotics Today* contains a Macrobiotic Resources Network that lists macrobiotic people and businesses that can be of help to you. Membership in the George Ohsawa Macrobiotic Foundation is also available. Membership includes a subscription and a discount on book purchases. Information on membership is included in the catalog and on the Foundation's website: *www. ohsawamacrobiotics.com.*

There are an increasing number of macrobiotic camps and conferences that can be an excellent source of macrobiotic learning. One of the best is the French Meadows Summer Camp held each summer in the Tahoe National Forest in California. Full information about the camp is in the catalog and on the website. A list of the major national mail-order suppliers completes catalog.

If you prefer to write for full information, send your request to:

George Ohsawa Macrobiotic Foundation
P. O. Box 3998
Chico, CA 95927-3998
Or, fax 530-566-9768

Other Books from the
George Ohsawa Macrobiotic Foundation

Acid Alkaline Companion - Carl Ferré; 2009; 121 pp; $15.00

Acid and Alkaline - Herman Aihara; 1986; 121 pp; $9.95

As Easy As 1, 2, 3 - Pamela Henkel and Lee Koch; 1990; 176 pp; $6.95

Basic Macrobiotic Cooking, 20th Anniversary Edition - Julia Ferré; 2007; 275 pp; $17.95

Basic Macrobiotics - Herman Aihara; 1998; 198 pp; $17.95

Book of Judo - George Ohsawa; 1990; 150 pp; $14.95

Calendar Cookbook - Cornellia Aihara; 1979; 160 pp; $24.95

Cancer and the Philosophy of the Far East - George Ohsawa; 1981; 165 pp; $14.95

Cooking with Rachel - Rachel Albert; 1989; 328 pp; $12.95

Essential Ohsawa - George Ohsawa, edited by Carl Ferré; 1994; 238 pp; $12.95

French Meadows Cookbook - Julia Ferré; 2008; 275 pp; $17.00

Macrobiotics: An Invitation to Health and Happiness - George Ohsawa; 1971; 128 pp; $11.95

Naturally Healthy Gourmet - Margaret Lawson with Tom Monte; 1994; 232 pp; $14.95

Philosophy of Oriental Medicine - George Ohsawa; 1991; 153 pp; $14.95

Unique Principle - George Ohsawa; 1973; 128 pp; $14.95

Zen Cookery - G.O.M.F.; 1985; 140 pp; $17.00

Zen Macrobiotics, Unabridged Edition - George Ohsawa, edited by Carl Ferré; 1995; 206 pp; $9.95

A complete selection of macrobiotic books is available from the George Ohsawa Macrobiotic Foundation, P.O. Box 3998, Chico, California 95965; 530-566-9765. Order toll free: (800) 232-2372. Or, see *www.ohsawamacrobiotics.com* for all books and PDF downloads of many books.

CPSIA information can be obtained at www.ICGtesting.com
Printed in the USA
BVOW072243241111

276755BV00001B/14/P